D1795896

The Child with a Chronic Medical Problem – Cardiac Disorders, Diabetes, Haemophilia

THE LIBRARY
NATIONAL FO[illegible] FOR
EDU[illegible]
IN[illegible]
TH[illegible]
SLO[illegible]
DATE: 2. 6. 86
CLASS: 2E, JGK
AUTHOR:
DINNAGE, R

B 1 251061 0

National Children's Bureau Bibliographies

3

The Child with a Chronic Medical Problem – Cardiac Disorders, Diabetes, Haemophilia

Rosemary Dinnage

NFER-NELSON

Published by the NFER-NELSON Publishing Company Ltd.,
Darville House, 2 Oxford Road East,
Windsor, Berkshire SL4 1DF, England.

and in the United States of America by

NFER-NELSON, 242 Cherry Street, Philadelphia,
PA 19106–1906.
Tel: (215) 238 0939. Telex: 244489.

First Published 1986
© 1986 National Children's Bureau

Library of Congress Cataloging in Publication data
Dinnage, Rosemary.
The child with a chronic medical problem – cardiac disorders, diabetes, haemophilia.

Includes index.
1. Chronic diseases in children – Psychological aspects. 2. Chronic diseases in children – Social aspects. 3. Heart – Abnormalities – Psychological aspects. 4. Diabetes in children – Psychological aspects. 5. Hemophilia in children – Psychological aspects. 6. Chronically ill children – Medical care – Psychological aspects. 7. Chronically ill children – Family relationships. 8. Chronically ill children – Education. I. Title. [DNLM: 1. Chronic Disease – in infancy & childhood. 2. Chronic Disease – psychology. 3. Diabetes Mellitus, Insulin-Dependent – psychology. 4. Heart Defects, Congenital – psychology. 5. Hemophilia – psychology. WS 200 D585c]
RJ380.D56 1986 618.92 85–28470
ISBN 0–7005–1013–3

All rights reserved, including translation. No part of this publication may be reproduced or transmitted in any form or by any means, electronic or mechanical, including photocopying, recording or duplication in any information storage and retrieval system, without permission in writing from the publishers.

Photoset by David John (Services) Ltd, Maidenhead

Printed in Great Britain by Henry Ling Ltd., at the Dorset Press, Dorchester, Dorset

ISBN 0–7005–1013–3
Code 8203 02 1

Contents

		Page
Acknowledgements		*vi*
Introduction		*vii*
SECTION I	Emotional and Social Adjustment	1
SECTION II	Family Adjustment	27
SECTION III	Educational Attainments	43
SECTION IV	General	59
Author index		69

Acknowledgements

Thanks are due first to the Department of Health and Social Security whose grant made this review possible.

The National Children's Bureau librarians, Ian Vallender and Biddy Cunnell, provided invaluable help in searching for references and obtaining books and photocopies. The librarian of the Tavistock Centre, Margaret Walker, was most helpful in providing further references by means of a computer scan.

The Chest and Heart Association, British Diabetic Association and Haemophilia Society were also kind enough to supply references.

In particular, thanks are due to Professor Catherine Peckham, who helped by discussing the medical aspects of the literature.

Finally, Doria Pilling, author of these booklets in their first edition, is not only responsible for part of the contents but has kindly advised on this updated version.

Introduction

In 1972–73 the National Children's Bureau published a series of concise research review booklets on childhood handicaps. Non-medical studies were summarized, and a brief overview added. In the years since, a great deal of further research and discussion has been published, and the Bureau felt it would be useful to have updated versions. The new booklets, therefore, contain material that was in the originals, together with more recent entries; and the reviews prefacing the annotated bibliographies have been rewritten.

The present booklet is concerned with research on the welfare of children with three chronic medical disorders – cardiac disorders, diabetes and haemophilia. These have very different clinical manifestations and prognoses, and differ in type and timing of medical treatment. Nevertheless these disorders have often been grouped together under various terms, most commonly as 'chronic illnesses' but also as 'chronic medical problems' or 'special health problems'. Children with these conditions require medical supervision greater than normal parental care and the disorders are potentially (though often remotely) life-threatening. The emphasis on modern management of all three conditions is on allowing the child to live a normal life. A number of other disorders might well have been included in the booklet but it was decided to concentrate on the three for which a reasonable amount of research is available.

SECTION I

Emotional and Social Adjustment

A recent careful study carried out in the Isle of Wight suggests that there is only a slightly higher rate of psychiatric disorder among physically handicapped children without neurological abnormalities than there is among non-handicapped children (Graham and Rutter, 1970). Disabilities of the children studied included heart conditions, diabetes and various types of orthopaedic disorders. There was no evidence of any greater risk of psychiatric disorder for any particular kind of handicap. Nevertheless each of the three disorders with which this review is concerned, cardiac defects, diabetes and haemophilia, has many distinctive features, so that the research literature on rates, type and determinants of psychiatric disorder in each needs to be examined separately.

Cardiac Disorders

Investigation of the emotional life of the child with a cardiac handicap is less straightforward than in the case of diabetes or haemophilia: cardiac malformation may sometimes be accompanied by other congenital handicaps, and, in addition, the effects of surgery – both benign and temporarily traumatizing – have to be taken into account. It is also relevant that over the years covered by this survey heart surgery has greatly changed and advanced.

Studies of children in this group have therefore been chiefly medically orientated, or have concentrated on the possibility of intellectual impairment. Interest in emotional and social development has been less pronounced. General articles (see Section IV) by Cooper (1959), Linde (1982), and Linde and Linde (1973), indicate the kind of problems that may be associated with cardiac disorder: early difficulties in feeding, parental anxiety, a sense of being 'different'. Kitchen (1978) has suggested that the phrase 'bad heart' has puzzling connotations for the child.

What little evidence exists is fairly evenly divided on the question of whether there are lasting emotional ill-effects. An early study by Neuhaus (1958) found children with cardiac illness to have a higher score for neurosis on several tests than healthy children. Garson *et al.* (1974) tested young people on a personality inventory some years after they had had successful heart surgery in childhood and found a significantly high number rating as 'neurotic'; the personality profile that emerged showed inclinations towards being sheltered, dependent, and impulsive. Neither of these studies is concerned with children operated on in more recent years, with recent techniques. Reed (1959), on the other hand, on the basis of clinical assessment rather than structured tests, assessed 'cardiac children' as being anxious and eager to please but no more maladjusted than their control group of normal children. Linde *et al.* (1966) based their conclusions on mothers' reports and found that children with a cardiac defect showed much the same level of emotional adjustment as two control groups.

It is possible that the rate of psychiatric disorder has changed in children with heart defects over recent years with the advances in surgical treatment. One of the major studies, carried out in Finland (Landtman *et al.*, 1960, 1968), found a marked decrease in behaviour problems (as seen by the mother) of children awaiting surgical correction. They were much commoner in the children seen in 1955–59 than in those seen in 1965–68. The authors considered that the main reason for the decrease was the improvement in mother–child relationships over the same period, owing to growing confidence in cardiac surgery.

If there are psychological ill-effects, there is some consensus that they are not related to the severity of the handicap but simply to its presence and to the family climate of anxiety. In the Finnish study, Landtman and his co-authors (1968) found that improvement in the child's mental health after operation was significantly related to improvement in the mother's attitude, which before operation had been rated as over-protective in a large number of cases. Further evidence comes from a part of their study which concerns 56 children who had been wrongly diagnosed as having a heart defect. The emotional reactions of these children and their mothers were very similar to those who really did have defects, and these improved when they were told that the diagnosis was wrong; the clear implication is that awareness of illness has a more powerful effect than any physical symptoms. Offord and Aponte (1967) and Offord *et al.* (1972) found, among a small group of children attending a cardiac clinic, that children with definite symptoms showed no more maladjustment than those without symptoms; the mother's perception of the gravity of the illness, whether accurate or not, had the determining effect on the quality of family life and on restrictions surrounding the child (see Section II). The same point emerges from part of the findings of Linde *et al.* (1966) in their study of a much larger group: maternal attitudes were a more important determinant of the children's adjustment than the severity of the defect, and these attitudes and anxieties were not necessarily determined by its severity.

There remains the question of the effect of cardiac surgery on children's health, intelligence, and emotional well-being. Recent studies have focused particularly on intellectual status after deep hypothermia and circulatory arrest (see pp.54, 56–7). Health, energy, appetite and sleep were found in the Landtman studies (1960, 1968) to be improved after surgery, as might be expected, and this is confirmed by the follow-up of a large group carried out by Bayer and Honzik (1976, see Section III) and by Boon (1972, see Section II) in this country. Emotional well-being was part of this general improvement. Bayer and Honzik found only transient negative reactions to being hospitalized for surgery, but there is evidence that it can also be traumatizing, as discussed by Linde and Linde (1973). Aisenberg *et al.* (1973) found that the children they studied, especially in the youngest age group, had a strong reaction against cardiac catheterization. Some indications of how fear of operations can be mitigated is suggested by Gabriel and Danilowicz's report (1978) of a programme of psychological preparation for surgery.

Haemophilia

There is rather more material on the psychological adjustment of haemophiliac children, but here again it is relevant to remember that there have been improvements in treatment during the years covered here; some of the studies using adolescents or young adults refer back to a time when treatment was less successful. Again, here, more interest has been shown in intelligence, school attendance, and employment than in emotional life.

Haemophilia can vary from a mild to a severe disability, and, as might be expected, the overall conclusions of Katz's (1963) research on over 1000 haemophiliacs in the United States are that the severely handicapped were less able to live a normal and successful life. Some of the mildly handicapped, however, also led very restricted lives; these were the subjects who lacked confidence and self-esteem. Several studies (Agle, 1964; Mattson and Gross, 1966; Madden *et al.*, 1982 (see Section II)) suggest that family influences are the most important determinants of mental health for haemophiliacs, as for the 'cardiac children', since they can instil these positive qualities. Goldy and Katz (1963) compared young haemophiliacs who had good adjustment with those who had poor adjustment, and concluded that anxious over-protection by mothers, and – more importantly – by fathers, was the crucial factor disrupting good mental health. They stress the dilemma of parents who have to make sure that a certain amount of caution is taken over physical activities and yet avoid over-protection. The way in which this dilemma is resolved has a considerable influence on the child's adjustment.

Results of studies assessing the actual extent of maladjustment are mixed. Grobler (1981) compared adolescent haemophiliacs with a matched control group and found no difference on three measures of emotional adjustment; Steinhausen (1976) also found no overall adjustment differences between a haemophiliac and a normal group in Germany. Out of 135 adolescent or young adult haemophiliacs, Bronks and Blackburn (1968) report that only 4.5 per cent had been treated by a psychiatrist, a figure which the authors indicate is not significantly higher than in the general population (see Section III).

On the other hand, Browne *et al.'s* (1960) study, based on Rorschach tests, suggests a certain amount of maladjustment, as do the results of projective tests administered to haemophiliac boys by Olch (1971a). In a small group studied by Salk *et al.* (1972, see Section II), 63 per cent were considered by their parents to have adapted to their illness, while Mattson and Gross (1966) assessed 77 per cent of their sample as having done so. Where relating maladjustment to severity of illness is concerned, there are contradictory conclusions from two studies: Steinhausen (1976) found severer handicaps to be associated with greater neuroticism, while Madden *et al.* (1982) found no such link. When haemophiliac boys do show maladjustment, there is some agreement that the commonest pattern is to be defiant and take unnecessary risks in reaction against the restrictions of their life (Agle, 1964; Mattson and Gross, 1966; Meijer, 1980 (see Section II)). Agle also found, in a small sample, some anxiety and depression in half of the children.

It is clear that the haemophiliac's bleeding episodes are not always due to a fall, bang, or cut; some appear to occur spontaneously. Several authors have found that stress or emotional disturbance may precipitate these spontaneious bleedings (Agle, 1964; Garlinghouse and Sharp, 1968; Salk *et al.*, 1972), although the physiological mechanism through which this occurs is not clear. Anticipation of events, either exciting or stressful, such as outings, hospital visits, or the start of school, are particularly liable to trigger spontaneous bleeding.

Diabetes

There has been a much greater interest in the emotional adjustment of diabetic children, especially over the past ten years or so. Investigators have been especially interested in the role of stress, particularly family stress, in provoking the onset of the illness and in upsetting control of it. Several recent review articles (Greydanus and Hoffmann, 1979; Hauser and Pollets, 1979; Kosub and Cerreto, 1981; Fisher *et al.*, 1982) summarize this material in more detail than there is space for here (see Section IV).

Since diabetes is not a congenital handicap like a heart defect or haemophilia and since its onset remains a puzzle, authors with an interest in psychosomatics have postulated both a 'pre-diabetic personality' and an important role for stress in triggering the illness. Stein and Charles (1971) found that 69 per cent of adolescent diabetics attending a clinic in New York had suffered either severe family stress, or the loss of a parent through death or divorce, before diabetes was diagnosed. From California, Leaverton *et al.* (1980) report a rather similar finding, 42 per cent of a sample of diabetic children having lost a parent through death or divorce before the onset of the illness, as compared to 19 per cent in a control group; more than half the losses occurred before the child was five. In a later (1975) study, Stein and Charles suggest that the development of juvenile diabetes may date back to infancy; a depth study of eight diabetic children revealed early feeding and weight disturbances which might constitute a 'pre-diabetic' state. Treuting (1962), Greydanus and Hoffmann (1979), and Hauser and Pollets (1979) in their reviews tend to agree that stress may be a factor in precipitating the onset of the disease, or at the least in affecting its course once established.

Studies of the actual rate of maladjustment among children after the establishment of diabetes are as contradictory as they are for children with heart defects or haemophilia. A number of studies from the 1960s to the 1980s have concluded that there is no more maladjustment among such children than would be expected in any comparable group. Sterky (1963), in Sweden, found an equal rate of emotional disturbance, as assessed through interviews, in groups of diabetic and of normal children, although the diabetics who were disturbed had more symptoms than the disturbed non-diabetic children. In Edinburgh, Olatawura (1972) carried out interviews with parents and teachers of juvenile diabetics at one hospital and found no differences between them and comparison groups; however, the groups selected for comparison were children from the hospital's medical and surgical departments, who may have had some reasons to be disturbed themselves. Ahnsjö *et al.*, 1981 (see Section III), again in Sweden, carried out a number of tests on diabetic children and matched controls at the onset of illness and three years later, and found no overall differences apart from a realistic anxiety about health.

Another study finding normally healthy emotional adjustment in juvenile diabetes was carried out by Gath *et al.*, 1980 (see Section III); no significant amount of psychiatric disorder was detected in a group of 76 diabetics. Lavigne *et al.* (1982) had similar findings for the girls in their sample, but boys, as assessed by parents, showed rather more signs of emotional disturbance; the authors suggest that the restrictions of the diabetic's life are less compatible with boys' roles than with girls'. Simonds (1976/7, 1977), investigating factors relevant to physical control of diabetes, found no surplus of psychiatric diagnoses in the diabetic group; nor did Sullivan in studies of adolescent girls (1976, 1979).

There are four studies concluding that, on the contrary, diabetic children are in fact prone to emotional disturbance. The most careful is that of Swift *et al.* (1967), who found much more disturbance in diabetic children than in matched controls (50 per cent as opposed to 10 per cent). Psychological testing and evaluation was thorough, and it is difficult to say why the results are opposed to those of the studies already discussed. Two of the research reviews also come to opposite conclusions, Greydanus and Hoffmann (1979) concluding that the majority view on diabetics' maladjustment is the right one, and Hauser and Pollets (1979) that most studies have not been sensitive enough to distinguish the subtle ways in which diabetes affects emotional life. Dunn and Turtle (see Section IV) in their review of the 'diabetic personality' (1981) argue that children from summer camps for diabetics are not typical, and a number of Swift *et al.*'s group were from a camp.

An earlier study by Swift and Seidman (1964), carried out without a control group, also found a rather high proportion of disturbed diabetic children. Anxiety, oral preoccupation, poor 'body image', and dependency were the traits noted. Fällström (1974) concluded that his group of diabetic children in Sweden had more emotional problems than a control group, but it appears to have been unusual in containing a number of children with a poor early history and abnormal EEG records. Ten out of 28 diabetic subjects were found by Birkbeck *et al.* (1968) to have significant psychiatric disturbance, but again no control group was used for comparison. Anxiety was again one of the main symptoms; perhaps this is a realistic response to the illness rather than a psychiatric symptom. Several authors (LaHood, 1970; Greydanus and Hoffmann, 1979; Tattersall and Lowe, 1981) stress the extra problems arising for diabetics at adolescence (see Section IV); possibly the age distribution of subjects in conflicting studies might offer a clue to their findings.

A number of authors have been interested in the question of good or poor metabolic control of the diabetic state, and there is a general consensus that poor control is associated with emotional or family disturbance (Swift and Seidman, 1964; Swift *et al.*, 1967; Birkbeck *et al.*, 1968; Ludvigsson, 1977 (see Section III); Simonds, 1976/7 and 1977; Gath *et al.*, 1980 (see Section III)). Adolescents may in fact deliberately upset their medical regime as a sign of rebellion against its restrictions. Koski *et al.*, 1976 (see Section II) found that on following up a group of diabetics in Finland, those who had changed from having good to having poor control had had to deal with family problems such as death, divorce, and parents' illness. Only two studies disagree to any extent with this consensus: in a small group of children Tietz and Vidmar (1972) found poor control to be more associated with adolescence than with maladjustment; and Simonds *et al.* (1981), studying adolescents only, conclude that there are individual metabolic and genetic factors that must be taken into account.

There is some conflict, then, in the evidence about the rate of psychiatric disorder in all three conditions. It is not finally established for any of them that extent of disorder is very different from that in the general population. The authors of one study state: 'diabetes imposes an additional difficulty upon the child or adolescent in achieving normal life adjustment' (Swift and Seidman, 1964). This is also applicable to the child with a heart condition or haemophilia. Nevertheless it does seem that, despite all difficulties, a majority of children, at least, manage to cope well. Where there is maladjustment, it will focus on the specific difficulties that the illness imposes on the child.

Perhaps the outstanding finding of many studies of all three conditions is the importance of parental attitudes in the determination of the child's adjustment. While the influence of parent–child relationships on the child's emotional adjustment has been emphasized for many years, the research on cardiac conditions, haemophilia, and diabetes stresses this particularly forcibly. Parental adjustment will be discussed in more detail in the next section.

NEUHAUS, E.C. (1958) *Psychosomatic Medicine,* 20, 3, 181–6.

A personality study of asthmatic and cardiac children

Asthmatic children, children with cardiac defects, normal children and siblings of the chronically ill children, all aged between 8 and 14 years, were tested on the Rorschach, Brown Personality Inventory and Despert Fables. The cardiac children had a significantly greater total neurotic score and gave significantly more dependent responses than matched normal children. Significant differences were not found between asthmatic and cardiac children, or between the chronically ill children and their healthy siblings. Findings suggest that children with a chronic illness have an emotional pattern that differs from the normal. The similar personality pattern in the siblings may be due to constitutional factors or to the presence of a chronically ill child in the family.

REED, M.K. (1959) *Dissertation Abstracts,* 20, Part 1, 385.

The intelligence, social maturity, personal adjustment, physical development, and parent–child relationship of children with congenital heart disease

Fifty children with congenital heart disease, aged three to eight, attending a cardiac out-patient clinic, did not differ significantly from non-handicapped matched controls in intelligence (Binet scale), social maturity (Vineland scale) or personal adjustment (clinically assessed). The severity of the defect was not related to intelligence or social maturity, Subjective impressions suggested that the children with heart defects had greater social anxiety and perceptiveness and were more eager to please the examiner, while the non-handicapped children were more relaxed.

Mothers of girls with congenital heart defects scored significantly higher than mothers of the non-handicapped girls on scales of 'intrusiveness' and 'fostering dependency' (Parental Attitude Research Instrument), but there were no significant differences between the mothers of boys in the two groups. Most mothers of the cardiac children seemed to have made a fairly realistic adjustment, and to have made good use of the medical advice given at the clinic.

BROWNE, W.J., MALLY, M.A., and KANE, R.P. (1960) *American Journal of Orthopsychiatry,* 30, 7, 730–40.

Psychosocial aspects of hemophilia; a study of twenty-eight hemophilic children and their families

A study of the effects on the course of the illness of emotional factors and mother–child relationships. Twenty-eight haemophiliac children aged one to 16 attending a clinic in Pittsburgh were interviewed or observed, and their medical histories studied; parents were also interviewed.

Only a minority of bleeding episodes were apparently precipitated by injuries, although injuries were more frequent on specific occasions, suggesting accident-proneness. Generally, spontaneous bleeding was more common, and appeared to show a seasonal variation, occurring most often at Christmas or other holiday times or whenever the child was anticipating some activity or increased independence. Personality patterns as assessed by Rorschach tests indicated conflict and aggression underlying docility. Parents reacted to the diagnosis of haemophilia with anxiety and unhappiness, and mothers felt particular guilt at being carriers of the disease, which seemed to result in more over-protectiveness than is found in mothers of children with other handicaps.

LANDTMAN, B., VALANNE, E.H., PENTTI, R., and AUKEE, M. (1960) *Annnales Paediatriac Fenniae,* 6, Supplement 15.

Psychosomatic behaviour of children with congenital heart disease. Pre- and post-operative studies of 84 cases

A study of the psychosomatic behaviour of 84 Finnish children with congenital heart disease, aged 5 to 17 years, before and after heart surgery. The children represented socially a cross-section of the Finnish population. The child's closest relative (mothers in 74 cases) was interviewed by the medical social worker on the child's admission to hospital; all the children were given a battery of psychological tests when they were awaiting the operation. Follow-up studies were carried out three months and one year after the operation.

Improvements in exercise tolerance (63 children), appetite (47), sleep habits (42), and susceptibility to infections (48) were found after the operation. Cardiological studies showed that the results were good in all cases. After the operation 23 children increased in intelligence by more than ten points, while only four children decreased by this amount. Increase was not related to increase of exercise ability or oxygen supply to the brain. The greatest improvement was found in children whose behaviour and emotional environment also changed favourably. Personality traits were generally in the average range before the operation and did not change significantly afterwards. Before the operation, though, 36 children showed signs of stress proneness, but this disappeared or diminished after the operation. Before the operation 37 mothers were considered to be normal in their attitudes to the child, 25 over-protective and eight rejecting. After the operation no changes were found in the attitudes of mothers considered normal, but improvements occurred in 11 over-protective and four rejecting mothers.

ETZWILER, D.D. and SINES, L.K. (1962) *Journal of the American Medical Association,* 181, 304–8.

Juvenile diabetes and its management: family, social and academic implications

Medical, family, social and academic information about 72 diabetic children (aged six to 15), mainly from middle-income families, attending a summer camp, was obtained from parents, physicians, schoolteachers and camp counsellors. Mothers were found to play the major role in the management of the disease. Most children (88.7 per cent) took some part in urine testing but only a third were involved in administering the insulin. It is suggested that the child should not assume primary responsibility for the management of his or her illness until he or she has a good understanding of the condition. Knowledge of the illness (only 15 per cent of children and 33 per cent of parents could answer 14 out of 15 basic questions about diabetes) and management practices need to improve if the incidence of long-term complications is to be minimized.

TREUTING, T.F. (1962) *American Journal of Medical Sciences,* 244, 1, 131–47.

The role of emotional factors in the etiology and course of diabetes mellitus: a review of recent literature

Four areas are reviewed: (1) role of psychological factors in the aetiology of diabetes: the research suggests that sustained and chronic emotional conflict may be a factor in the onset of the illness; (2) role of psychological factors in the course of the illness: fluctuations in the course of diabetes have been found to be related to emotional factors, although exactly how and why is not known for certain. These changes are more important and frequent in juvenile diabetes; (3) attitudes and reactions produced by the illness: most researchers emphasize the uniqueness of diabetes amongst chronic illnesses, which may give rise to emotional problems and rebellion in young patients; (4) role of psychological factors in treatment: effective control of diabetes requires the cooperation of the patient, and the doctor needs to understand him or her as a person.

DANOWSKI, T.S. (1963) *Diabetes,* 12, 2, 183–4.

Emotional stress as a cause of diabetes mellitus

Reconsideration of the problem leads to the conclusion that emotional stress cannot cause diabetes in normal individuals but it may bring about clinical manifestations of the illness in those who have an inherent predisposition to diabetes.

GOLDY, F.B. and KATZ, A.H. (1963) *Children,* 10, 189–93.

Social adaptation in hemophilia

Findings from an investigation of 1100 adult haemophiliacs, carried out by the University of California. Forty subjects, representing those who had made relatively good or poor social adjustment, were interviewed to explore the relationship between early childhood experiences and later adjustment. Subjects generally felt that their mothers had been over-protective whether or not the mothers knew they were carriers of the disease. Over-protection, though, was accepted from mothers but not from fathers. The key factor in the haemophiliac's social competence was the attitude of the father – 'good adjusters' had fathers who were permissive or indifferent while 'poor adjusters' were over-protected by both parents.

Whether the haemophiliacs felt themselves to be different from others depended not on severity of illness but on whether they had been allowed to take part in normal play. A large number of 'good adjusters' said that their parents had encouraged normal childhood activities while most of the 'poor adjusters' had experienced parental opposition. Subjects thought that parents of haemophiliac children should allow the children themselves to learn their own limits. Adolescence was often less difficult than earlier childhood for haemophiliacs because there were bases for social relationships other than physical activities. (See also Katz, 1963, below).

KATZ, A.H. (1963) *American Journal of Public Health,* 53, 10, 1966–75.

Social adaptation in chronic illness; a study of hemophilia

Findings from the questionnaire survey of 1055 haemophiliac adults from all over the United States are reported and discussed (see Goldy and Katz, 1963, for a report of the second part of this study). 76 per cent of the sample had experienced arthropathies (joint stiffening or haemophilic arthritis – the usual cause of disabilities among haemophiliacs) at some time, but only just over half had received rehabilitative care for them. About 6 per cent of the sample, generally, but by no means always, severely handicapped, had rarely or never worked. Such individuals also often had limited social participation and did not contemplate marriage. The author considers that they have never established a self-concept as a social competent individual who has a limiting condition of haemophilia; instead their self-concept is of a chronically handicapped person. Many haemophiliacs, though, have a strong drive towards as normal a social role as possible – in work, marriage and other social relationships.

49 per cent of the sample were or had been married. 52.1 per cent were employed – many in jobs involving physical work – 1.14 per cent were retired and 26.4 per cent still at school. The income level of those employed was similar to that in the general population. Among the measures recommended to help more haemophiliacs to lead satisfactory lives are parental counselling, early medical treatment to prevent impairments and earlier vocational counselling.

STERKY, G. (1963) *Acta Paediatrica* (Stockholm), 52, 377–90.

Family background and state of mental health in a group of diabetic schoolchildren

119 diabetic school children (aged 7 to 20), living in Stockholm, were paired with 119 non-diabetic children on the basis of sex, age, school class and employment of father; the children were observed over the period of a year during a number of physical examinations and their mothers were interviewed. A much higher rate of mental disturbance was found among the mothers of the diabetics (27.6 per cent) than among the mothers of the non-diabetic children (11.1 per cent), the most common disturbance in both groups being anxiety.

Among the children, mental disturbance was absent in as many diabetics (54.5 per cent) as non-diabetics (55.6 per cent). When diabetic children did show mental disturbance, however, they tended to have more symptoms than the mentally disturbed non-diabetic children. Emotional lability and difficulties with companions were found significantly more often among the mentally disturbed diabetic children than among the non-diabetic. Most of the mental disorders were mild, but five diabetics and one non-diabetic child had severe disorders. School achievements were similar in the diabetics and non-diabetics.

No connection was found between school achievement and age of onset of diabetes, duration or diabetic control. Diabetic children with mental disturbance were more likely than those without to have mentally disturbed mothers or poor diabetic control.

AGLE, D.P. (1964) *Archives of Internal Medicine,* 114, 76–82.

Psychiatric studies of patients with hemophilia and related states

A report of findings from psychiatric interviews with 16 subjects (13 with haemophilia, three with Christmas disease). All subjects felt a realistic fear of the bleeding, and resulting pain, immobility and separation from their families. Nine thought they had experienced extreme over-protection from their mothers (although the fathers often showed little interest in them). Not being allowed to take part in normal childhood activities had emphasized their feelings of difference from other children. Over-protection and fear of activity led to two extremes – recurrent risk-taking (seen in nine subjects) or passive-dependent behaviour (seen in two). In eight other cases subjects reported that their behaviour had changed from passive dependence to a more aggressive independence and that there had been a subsequent improvement in their clinical state.

It was also reported (by ten subjects) that episodes of spontaneous bleeding sometimes followed stressful emotional situations or the anticipation of them. The study suggests that psychological factors may affect the course of the illness. Counselling the parents so that they allow reasonable activities in childhood is recommended.

SWIFT, C.R. and SEIDMAN, F.L. (1964) *Journal of the American Academy of Child Psychiatry,* 3, 3, 500–15.

Adjustment problems in juvenile diabetes

Forty children and young adults (ages 2 to 20), referred by private physicians in the New Jersey area, were given a psychiatric interview and a battery of psychological tests; parents were interviewed by a psychiatric social worker.

62 per cent of the children were judged to be normal and 37.5 per cent to be pathological. Prominent features of the group were greater manifest anxiety than would be expected for age (in 52.5 per cent), greater latent anxiety (85 per cent), greater preoccupation with food (50 per cent), and a damaged or inadequate body image (55 per cent). While 40 per cent of the children were more dependent than would be expected for their age, 10 per cent were more independent. The social worker judged the emotional tone of the home to be good in 67.5 per cent of cases. Mothers' acceptance of the disease was realistic in 71.7 per cent of cases, but 48.7 per cent of mothers were considered over-protective and 10.3 per cent neglectful. Control of the diabetes was good in 37.5 per cent of cases and poor in 17.5 per cent. 52 per cent of the children showed good overall adjustment, 35 per cent fair and 12.5 per cent poor.

Control of diabetes was better in children who were classified as well adjusted, showed less anxiety and had a better body image, where the emotional tone of the home was good and the diabetes less and of shorter duration. The less severe the illness the better the adjustment. Socio-economic status was significantly related to overall adjustment and psychiatric evaluation. While the children had a high proportion of adjustment problems, the authors found also that many showed remarkable personality strengths; diabetes may give rise to difficulties in some susceptible children, but may accelerate maturity in others.

LINDE, L.M., RASOF, B., DUNN, O.J., and RABB, E. (1966) *Pediatrics,* 38, 1, 92–101.

Attitudinal factors in congenital heart disease

A comparison of the relationship between adjustment and parental attitudes in cardiac and normal children. Subjects were 98 children with a congenital heart defect and cyanosis, 100 children with a heart defect but no cyanosis, 81 healthy siblings of the cardiac children and 40 normal children.

The cardiac children were significantly lower in intelligence than both the groups of normal children. While intelligence was unrelated to the child's adjustment or maternal attitudes in the normal children there was some relationship between these three variables in the cardiac children. There was little difference between the cardiac and normal children (both groups) in level of adjustment, as assessed by mothers' reports. Maternal attitudes were a more important determinant of the cardiac child's adjustment than the degree of his or her incapacity. The presence of a heart condition in the child, rather than the severity of the defect, appeared to be the main determinant of maternal anxiety. Protectiveness and attention were much greater for the cardiac child than for his or her healthy sibling, the sibling receiving less than the other normal children. (See also Rasof *et al.,* 1967 (see Section III) and Linde *et al.,* 1970.)

MATTSON, A. and GROSS, S. (1966) *Journal of Pediatrics,* 68, 952–64.

Social and behavioral studies on hemophilic children and their families

Thirty-five haemophiliac boys, from 22 families, mainly in the middle socio-economic range, were given psychiatric interviews and were observed over a two-year period. Twenty-seven (77 per cent) were judged to be well adapted to their illness. They generally took as much part as possible in sports, cooperated well with parents and hospital staff during bleeding episodes and had a basic understanding of their illness. Mothers of these children were able to make a good or satisfactory adjustment, despite anxiety or guilt. They were able to bring the children up with realistic restrictions, to cooperate with medical care and to explain the illness well. The majority of the fathers of the well-adapted children, in a few cases after an initial depression at the time of diagnosis, took an active part in the children's care. Three of the eight poorly-adapted children led restricted and dependent lives, having accepted the mother's over-protection, while the other five children showed recurrent risk-taking behaviour. The study emphasizes the relationship between parental acceptance of the disease and the adjustment of the child.

SWIFT, C.R., SEIDMAN, F.L., and STEIN, H. (1967) *Psychosomatic Medicine,* 29, 6, 555–71.

Adjustment problems in juvenile diabetes

Fifty-five diabetic children (from a summer camp, clinics and private medical practices in New Jersey) and 50 matched control children were each given a psychiatric evaluation and a battery of psychological tests; parents were interviewed at home.

Emotional disturbance was found much more frequently in the diabetic children (50 per cent) than in the controls (10 per cent). The diabetic children were found to be significantly more abnormal in dependence–independence balance, self-percepts, manifest and latent anxiety, sexual identification, hostility expression and oral preoccupation. The adjustment of the diabetic children to home and peers was significantly worse than that of the non-diabetic children: while about two-thirds of the controls were making a good adjustment only one-quarter to one-third of the diabetic children were doing so. There were no significant differences in the school adjustment of the two groups.

The emotional atmosphere of the diabetic children's homes was poorer and mothers showed more extreme attitudes of protection or neglect. Diabetic control became worse as the duration of the illness increased, and was also worse in children with poorer emotional adjustment, lower IQ and family income and earlier onset of the illness. Self-percept and dependence–independence balance were related to the child's acceptance of the illness and the emotional atmosphere of the home.

WEIL, W.B. Jr. and SUSSMAN, M.B. (1967) *American Journal of Diseases of Children,* 113, 454–60.

Social patterns and diabetic glucosuria

In an experiment at a summer camp for diabetic children it was found that groups of boys and girls, aged 9 to 12 years, increased their glucosuria (excretion of glucose in the urine) more during a period in which competitive sporting activities between groups were organized than would be expected under normal camp conditions. Children under the age of eight years, though, showed relatively little change in glucosuria during the competitive period. It would appear that younger children do not respond to any great extent to group activities and these have little effect on the stability of their diabetic control. Older children, in contrast, are affected by group activities and the less competitive these are the greater the stability of their diabetic control. Changes in glucosuria during the period of 'inter-group competition' were not related to the social adjustment of individual children.

BIRKBECK, J.A., KLONOFF, H., and MCTAGGART, A.H. (1968) *Diabetics,* Annual Meeting Supplement, 17, 317–8.

Emotional disturbance in juvenile diabetics

Twenty-eight adolescents (12 boys, 16 girls) with diabetes were interviewed in-depth by a psychiatrist and given a battery of psychological tests; parents were also interviewed in-depth. The average intelligence was 118, significantly above normal (Wechsler Intelligence scale). Ten subjects (nine girls, one boy) showed evidence of significant psychiatric disturbance. There was a strong relationship between poor diabetic control and emotional disturbance. In general, subjects showed productivity, organizational ability, wide interests and effective responses, but also many features of anxiety. On the Minnesota Multiphasic Personality Inventory 38 per cent of parents showed signs of overt disturbance.

GARLINGHOUSE, J. and SHARP, L.J. (1968) *Nursing Research,* 17, 1, 32–7.

The hemophilic child's self-concept and family stress in relation to bleeding episodes

This study found a slight relationship between family stress (as reported by the mother) and the number of spontaneous bleeding episodes experienced by a haemophiliac child. A slight relationship was also found between the strength of the child's self-concept and the number of bleeding episodes. This relationship only held, though, when stresses were low. When stresses were high they tended to be associated with more bleeding episodes regardless of the strength of the child's self-concept. Subjects were 18 haemophiliac children (mainly aged 9 to 14), attending a haemophilia centre in Seattle, Washington.

LANDTMAN, B., VALANNE, E.H., and AUKEE, M. (1968) *Annales Paediatriae Fenniae,* 14, 3, 71–92.

Emotional implications of heart disease. A study of 256 children with real and with 'imaginary' heart disease

A further study of the emotional adjustment of children operated on for congenital heart disease at the Children Hospital in Helsinki (see also Landtman *et al.,* 1960). Subjects were 200 children with congenital heart defects (164 acyanotic, 36 cyanotic), including the 84 children from the original study.

Time of waiting for the operation was more than five years in 111 cases. One year after the operation all the cardiac children were able to lead normal or practically normal lives. In the cardiac children no relationship was found between the severity of the defect and the mother's attitude, the child's behaviour before the operation, or the child's intelligence. Behaviour of the children, though, was related to the mothers' attitudes. Improvements in attitudes occurred in 47 of the mothers considered to be over-protective (61) or rejecting (9) before the operation. Improvements were also found in the behaviour of 80 of the 133 children considered normal before the operation and in 24 of the 67 emotionally disturbed children. Thirty of the children increased in IQ more than ten points after the operation, while only six decreased in IQ by this amount.

Two years after the operation teachers reporting on the behaviour and progress of 104 of the children found improvements in almost three-quarters.

A study was also made of the emotional adjustment of 56 children who had been mistakenly diagnosed as having a heart defect, all of whom had subjective symptoms of heart complaint. Emotional reactions of the children with imaginary heart disease and their mothers were very similar to those found in children who actually had heart disease. Behaviour of the children improved in 35 cases after they were told they had a normal heart, symptoms disappeared in 42 cases and the IQ of four children improved by ten or more points. School reports of these children were generally above average both before and after they were found to be free of heart disease.

GRAHAM, P. and RUTTER, M. (1970) In: RUTTER, M., TIZARD, J. and WHITMORE, K. (Eds) *Education, Health and Behaviour.* London: Longman, 309–27.

Psychiatric aspects of physical disorder

In a survey of handicapped children on the Isle of Wight, 10- to 12-year-old children with physical disorders (orthopaedic, heart disease, diabetes and other disorders) were found to have only a slightly higher rate of psychiatric problems (10.5 per cent), as judged from a parental questionnaire, than the general population (6.8 per cent) (difference only bordered on statistical significance). Findings were similar on a teachers' questionnaire. While significantly more of the children with physical disorders felt miserable or had frequent headaches compared with the general population, rates of other behaviour difficulties were similar in the two groups.

KATZ, A.H. (1970a) Chapter 4 in *Haemophilia. A Study in Hope and Reality.* Springfield, Illinois: Charles C. Thomas.

The haemophiliac's family: a total involvement

A review of research by the author himself and by others of the emotional problems of the haemophiliac boy and his parents. The author concludes that, on the whole, his research shows that most haemophiliacs and their families have done very well, without having received much professional help or counselling – but if such help were available they could do even better and could avoid much distress.

KRONES, P.D. (1970) *Dissertation Abstracts International,* 30, 8-B, 3870–1.

Level of aspiration and the evaluation of self and others by diabetic and non-diabetic children

Forty-four children, aged 10 to 16, attending a summer camp for diabetic children, and 44 non-handicapped schoolchildren in the same age range, were administered a level of aspiration task and a questionnaire designed to evaluate self-concept. Significantly more of the diabetic than of the non-diabetic children were found to overestimate or underestimate their ability on the level of aspiration task – indicating that diabetic children have negative feelings about themselves more frequently than non-diabetic children.

LINDE, L.M., RASOF, B., and DUNN, O.J. (1970) *Acta Paediatrica Scandinavica,* 59, 2, 169–176.

Longitudinal studies of intellectual and behavioural development in children with congenital heart disease

The final report of a series of studies over a five-year period comparing the intelligence and adjustment of children with cyanotic and acyanotic heart disease and normal children (see also Linde *et al.,* 1966; Rasof *et al.,* 1967 (see Section III)).

During this period more than 40 per cent of the cardiac children underwent operations, and the present study compares the development of operated and non-operated children.

All groups made some gains in mean IQ, but the only change that reached statistical significance was in the operated cyanotic group. Initial low IQ in the cyanotic children can be attributed, at least in part, to their incapacity and the IQ increment to clinical improvement following the operation. Acyanotic children were less handicapped and nearer to their true potential and, therefore, less change occurred whether or not they were operated upon. As with intellectual change, the greatest improvement in adjustment and behaviour occurred in the operated cyanotic group. The non-operated cyanotic group showed a significant decline in general adjustment, while both the operated and non-operated acyanotic groups showed no change.

Mothers of operated children, cyanotic and acyanotic, decreased in anxiety and pampered their children less during the study period. Mothers of the non-operated acyanotic children also decreased in protectiveness, probably due to the decline in symptoms in the group with age.

DEL VECCHIO, F.A. (1971) *Dissertation Abstracts International,* 32, 2-B, 1208.

A comparative study of selected personality variables in diabetic and non-diabetic children

Previous research has suggested that diabetic children are more constricted than non-handicapped children. The present study compared two possible manifestations of constriction – level of anxiety and creative ability – in 50 diabetic children (aged 7 to 16) living in New Jersey, and 50 matched control children. The two groups showed no overall differences in creative ability. However, some evidence that the diabetic children were more anxious was found.

OLCH, D. (1971a) *Journal of Personality Assessment,* 35, 1, 72–9.

Personality characteristics of hemophiliacs

Forty-five haemophiliacs from Seattle, Washington (see also Olch, 1971b (Section III)) were administered a number of projective tests (Rorschach, Draw-a-Person, and making up stories to four verbal cues). Personality characteristics resembled those that have been reported for diabetics and asthmatics. Nevertheless a single typical haemophiliac personality was not found – individuals reacted to and coped with the illness in many different ways.

STEIN, S.P. and CHARLES, E.S. (1971) *American Journal of Psychiatry,* 128, 6, 700–4.

Emotional factors in juvenile diabetes mellitus: a study of early life experience of adolescent diabetics

This study suggests that some individuals are physiologically susceptible to diabetes and that psychological stress, such as parental loss or severe family disturbance may lead to the disease becoming clinically manifest. 69 per cent of adolescent diabetics, from a lower socio-economic level background, attending the diabetic clinic at the Bronx Hospital Municipal Centre, had suffered parental loss (due to separation, divorce or death) or severe family disturbance (severe physical or mental illness of a parent or intense marital discord), compared with 19 per cent of the control subjects – adolescents with hereditary blood disorders, from a similar social background, attending another clinic at the Hospital Centre. 77 per cent of the diabetics had suffered the parental losses before the disease was clinically diagnosed.

OLATAWURA, M.O. (1972) *African Journal of Medical Science,* 3, 231–40.

The psychiatric complications of diabetes mellitus in children

Fifty diabetic children from an Edinburgh clinic were compared with 50 matched children from the same hospital who had been newly referred to medical, surgical, or ENT departments. Home interviews with mothers, with a precoded behaviour inventory, were carried out by the author, and questionnaires were completed by the children's teachers. There were no significant differences between the groups, except that the control children were more liable to sleep disturbance and to stealing. These results may be partly due to the management policy of the clinic.

TIETZ, W. and VIDMAR, J.T. (1972) *Psychiatry in Medicine,* 3, 1, 67.

The impact of coping styles on the control of juvenile diabetes

In this study of 21 children with diabetes, from a lower socio-economic level background (15 from minority ethnic groups), no correlation was found between the degree of control of diabetes and its duration, knowledge of diabetes, number of siblings, intactness of family, degree of psychopathology, intelligence of the child or parents, birth rank, ethnic group or social class. A relationship between good control and a family history of diabetes was found. A number of those with only fair or poor control appeared to be in the midst of an adolescent growth spurt, suggesting that biological factors may play a part in control. The onset of diabetes had a great impact on all the families. The initial shock was followed by a basic anxiety that the child might die. This fear was often partially repressed but persisted on a preconscious or conscious level. It is suggested that the family style of coping with this fear affects the degree of control achieved. The argument is illustrated with case studies.

AISENBERG, R.B., WOLFF, P.H., ROSENTHAL, A., and NADAS, A.S. (1973) *Pediatrics,* 51, 1051–9.

Psychological impact of cardiac catheterization

A study to determine the extent of psychological disturbances in young cardiac patients after catheterization. Fifty children between 4 and 15 in Boston, with a variety of cardiac handicaps, were divided into three age groups: 4- to 6-year-olds, 6- to 12-year-olds, and 12- to 16-year-olds. Children with central nervous system disorders and the acutely ill had been excluded, together with all children who had been catheterized previously, and all with post-catheterization complications. The catheterization was carried out under Demerol in a darkened room; most children slept a certain amount during the procedure. Afterwards, nurses and the play specialist filled out behaviour observation forms concerning eating, sleeping, crying, and parents' reports. The play specialist recorded play behaviour before and after catheterization. Interviews were carried out with each child and parent a few weeks before and after the procedure, and intelligence tests and several projective tests administered.

It was found that 70 per cent of the children responded negatively to their experience, with aggression, emotional changes, and behavioural regression. They were afraid of being left alone, and showed increased anxiety on the projective tests. This was true of 93 per cent in the youngest group, 71 per cent in the middle group, and 43 per cent in the older group. The authors conclude that cardiac catheterization is not a psychologically innocuous procedure, especially for very young children, and may even have long-term harmful results. Children should be thoroughly prepared for the event, and parents encouraged to spend as much time as possible with younger patients.

FÄLLSTRÖM, K. (1974) *Acta Paediatrica Scandinavica,* Supplement 251.

On the personality structure in diabetic schoolchildren aged 7–15 years

Personality development in all 59 diabetic children aged 7 to 15 attending a clinic in Göteborg, Sweden, was studied, together with a matched group of controls. Thirteen of the diabetic children had had perinatal complications such as low birthweight, forceps delivery, or asphyxia. The assessment comprised an intelligence test, a series of projective tests, interviews with the children, their parents, and teachers, and an EEG investigation.

The children's intelligence was above average. The projective tests suggested that the diabetic children had a number of emotional problems as compared to the controls, and a disturbed body image, though only three of them needed professional help. Emotional lability was related to early onset of the illness, long duration, and hypoglycaemic convulsions. Cerebrolesional traits and perceptual disturbances were also common in the diabetic children, and these were positively correlated with hypoglycaemic convulsions and unusual EEG records. Five children had definitely abnormal EEG records, which were associated with frequent hospitalizations, convulsions, and low birthweight. Emotional symptoms in the diabetic children are considered to be partly a reaction to their life situation, but also related to disturbances of basic processes (development of body image, ego structure, and identification), and to cerebrolesional and perceptual disturbances.

GARSON, M.D., WILLIAMS, R.B., and RECKLESS, J. (1974) *Behavioural Pediatrics*, 85, 3, 429–33.

Long-term follow-up of patients with tetralogy of Fallot: Physical health and psychopathology

To assess possible effects in young adults who had recovered from congenital heart disease, 37 young people with an average age of 19 who had been symptom-free for several years were tested (nearly a third of the original group as traced had died). 92 per cent of the 37 had had an operation in childhood, 51 per cent two operations, 8 per cent three; average age at first surgery had been 6.9 years. Cattell's 16 PF Personality Inventory was administered to the group and 'neuroticism' scores extracted; 22 out of 37 rated as neurotic, as opposed to an expected average of seven. Five neurosis factors were extracted from the scores: weak superego, being dependent, being over-protected, being less than well informed, and operating on the basis of feeling rather than thought. When subjects were scored for severity of symptoms from their case records, neurosis was associated with less severe symptoms, but also with more hospitalization. Reasons for the results are discussed: organic causes were unlikely, as the group was of normal intelligence, and hospitalization and family attitudes are considered more relevant.

STEIN, S.P. and CHARLES, E.S. (1975) *Psychosomatic Medicine,* 37, 237–44.

Emotional factors in juvenile diabetes mellitus: A study of the early life experiences of eight diabetic children

The developmental history of eight diabetic children aged 13 to 18 was studied in depth and compared with that of their siblings. Data were collected by long interviews and from hospital records containing material from before the onset of diabetes, and were recorded on questionnaires and a medical history form. The results showed, in the children who later developed diabetes, higher birthweight, early feeding difficulties, dependency on the mother, and difficulties during delivery. Case histories are given. The authors suggest that the aetiology of the 'oral-dependent' personality described in the literature on juvenile diabetes may be rooted in early childhood. Theories about a 'pre-diabetic' state are discussed, and related to the disturbances of appetite and weight present in the early life of the diabetic children.

STEINHAUSEN, H.C. (1976) *Journal of Psychosomatic Research,* 20, 5, 461–7.

Hemophilia: a psychological study in chronic disease in juveniles

Fifty haemophiliac boys in Hamburg were matched for age, sex, and sibling order with control children. Questionnaire tests of intelligence, extraversion, neuroticism and aggression were administered to all the children, and no significant differences were found between the two groups; severer handicap, however, was associated with greater neuroticism and less extraversion. The haemophiliac group also answered a questionnaire about perceived parental behaviour. Few perceived mothers as over-protective, and those who did were the more severely handicapped children. Reasons for differences between the results of this and previous studies are discussed.

SIMONDS, J.F. (1976/7) *International Journal of Psychiatry in Medicine,* 7, 2, 133–151.

Psychiatric status of diabetic youth in good and poor control

In an attempt to find out whether children with poor diabetic control were more disturbed than those with good control, 80 children of six and over from a clinic in Missouri were studied. All children had been rated for diabetic control, and two matched groups with good and poor control were arranged. Socio-economic status was found to be similar in the two groups. The children's psychiatric status was evaluated by the author on the basis of a 40-minute interview and a checklist filled in by mothers. Six children (7.5 per cent of the total) were rated as psychiatric problems, most of them pre-pubertal girls. This was no higher than might be expected in the general population. A significantly greater number of patients with poor control, however, were considered to have interpersonal conflicts.

SIMONDS, J.F. (1977) *Diabetes,* 26, 921–5.

Psychiatric status of diabetic youth matched with a control group

The author assessed three groups of children and young people for signs of psychiatric disorder, at a semi-structured interview: 40 diabetics in good control and 40 in poor control from a Missouri clinic, and 40 healthy control children. The good-control group had significantly fewer conflicts than the other two groups, and the poor-control group showed most signs of anxiety and depression. Nevertheless, psychiatric diagnoses were made with equal frequency – which was low – in all three groups.

GABRIEL, H.P. and DANILOWICZ, D. (1978) *British Heart Journal,* 40, 1046–51.

Postoperative responses in 'prepared' child after cardiac surgery

Fifty children and adolescents in New York, who had had cardiac operations, were studied. All had been given special preparation for surgery: they visited the ward in advance, and had talks with hospital staff. Younger children were given a shared room with a parent. Once admitted to the hospital, they were shown the recovery room and intensive care unit, and equipment such as masks, catheters, and oxygen tents. Parents were asked to be present before the child went into the theatre and after he or she woke in the recovery room. They were told to expect some behaviour changes in the children afterwards, and ensured easy access to advice. Three months after the operation a questionnaire regarding the child's behaviour was sent to the family. Negative reactions were very much more common in the under-sevens than at other ages; and 8- to 11-year-olds had more positive reactions than children who were either younger or older. By two months after the operation most of the negative reactions had disappeared; there was only one long-term reaction, in a child who had had unusually long and painful experiences.

KITCHEN, L.W. (1978) *Journal of Family Practice,* 6, 4, 777–83.

Psychological factors in congenital heart disease in children

A review of the literature on the subject, which concludes that (a) many children with congenital heart disease suffer from some degree of diminished self-esteem that is not necessarily related to the severity of the handicap; (b) the child's emotional adjustment is to some extent a function of maternal anxiety; (c) the mother's anxiety is unrelated to the severity of the heart disease; (d) cardiac catheterization may cause anxiety; (e) studies of the relationship between cognitive functioning and the illness have yielded conflicting results. It is recommended that the illness be talked about openly and that children be encouraged to explain what they feel a 'bad heart' means to them.

SULLIVAN, B.-J. (1978) *Diabetes Care,* 1, 1, 18–22.

Self-esteem and depression in adolescent diabetic girls

105 diabetic girls from a camp for diabetics in Massachusetts were compared with 100 non-diabetic girls from a suburban middle-class community. All were between 12 and 16, and were tested in self-rating inventories of depression and self-esteem; questions were also asked about social activities and sports. Self-esteem ratings showed only a non-significant trend for diabetics to have lower self-esteem, and in terms of their activities the groups were very similar. Comparison of depression inventories, however, showed that twice as many diabetic girls as controls experienced moderate or severe depression; but the increased scores were in the area of physical symptoms such as sleep and eating rather than pessimism and distress. It was concluded that the two groups were very similar, but that the diabetic girls were more aware of their physical states.

SULLIVAN, B.-J. (1979) *Psychosomatic Medicine,* 41, 2, 119–38.

Adjustment in diabetic adolescent girls: 1. Development of the Diabetic Adjustment Scale

A 37-item scale was designed to assess life adjustment in 105 adolescent girls at a camp for diabetics. It covered peer and family relationships, body image, dependence/independence, school adjustment, and attitudes towards diabetes. Preliminary results suggest that the questionnaire was answered honestly, that this group of girls was relatively well adjusted, and that their attitudes towards their illness correlated positively with measures of adjustment.

LEAVERTON, D.R., WHITE, C.A., MCCORMICK, C.R., PERRIN SMITH, M.S., and SHEIKHOLISLAM, B. (1980) *American Academy of Child Psychiatry* 19, 678–89.

Parental loss antecedent to childhood diabetes mellitus

The incidence of loss of a parent was documented for 121 diabetic children and 37 control children in California. For the diabetics, 42 per cent had lost a parent, nearly always through divorce, before the onset of the illness, as compared to 19 per cent of the controls. Diabetic children with parental loss and severe family disturbance had by far the greatest number of recurrent hospitalizations. More than half the losses occurred before the age of five, which suggests that early loss and its subsequent chronic stress may be important.

GROBLER, T. (1981) In: EGLI, H. and INWOOD, M.J. (Eds) *The Haemophiliac in the Eighties,* 259–61.

Personality, self-concept and vocational interest in a group of adolescent haemophiliacs

Comparing 40 adolescent haemophiliacs in South Africa with a control group, the author found no difference between the two groups on three measures of adjustment and ambition.

SIMONDS, J., GOLDSTEIN, D., WALKER, B., and RAWLINGS, S. (1981) *Diabetes Care,* 4, 6, 610–15.

The relationship between psychological factors and blood glucose regulation in insulin-dependent diabetic adolescents

Adolescent diabetics who were able to maintain good blood glucose regulation were compared with those with poor regulation in order to discover what personality variables distinguish the two groups. Fifty-two 13- to 19-year-olds, mainly middle-class in background, attending a centre in Missouri, were divided into those with adequate and those with inadequate regulation. Three self-reporting personality scales were completed by them, and in some cases mothers answered questions on management and behaviour. There were no significant differences between the groups in the personality variables or the mothers' reports, though those with poor regulation scored significantly higher on anxiety, were more likely to feel they were 'different', and more likely to break their diet when upset. Self-concept, in general, was quite positive. Results may have been influenced by the fact that subjects came from the same social background and were under the same medical regimen. Nevertheless, there are underlying metabolic and genetic factors which need to be considered when differentiating subjects according to the degree of blood glucose regulation.

LAVIGNE, J.V., TRAISMAN, H.S., MARR, T.J., and CHASNOFF, I.J. (1982) *Diabetes Care,* 5, 4, 420–6.

Parental perceptions of the psychological adjustment of children with diabetes and their siblings

A study of diabetic children, their siblings, and a control group of healthy children. The diabetics, aged 6 to 16, were all attending a private paediatric practice in Chicago and the controls were attending for routine check-ups. Socio-economic status was fairly high. Parents of all children completed inventories relating to children's behaviour and to marital adjustment. Diabetic boys of 6 to 11 showed rather more psychiatric symptoms than siblings or controls, but not girls; in the 12 to 16 age group the trend was repeated. No relation was found between symptoms and degree of diabetic control. It is suggested that the dependence and patience involved in diabetic care are less compatible with the male role than the female, and also that there may have been a class effect.

KINMONTH, A., LINDSAY, M.K.M., and BAUM, J.D. (1983) *British Medical Journal,* 286, 6369, 952–4.

Social and emotional complications in a clinical trial among adolescents with diabetes mellitus

Eleven adolescent diabetics who were taking part in an experiment on diet had been specially chosen for maturity, family stability, and informed consent to the research. The article shows that unexpected difficulties can nevertheless arise: one child experienced severe family stress, two became distressed by the blood testing procedures, one admitted cheating on the diet, one reacted by his diabetes becoming uncontrollable, several developed school problems. Such problems should be borne in mind in planning future research on diabetes; both better selection and more support during the experience are recommended.

SECTION II

Family Adjustment

Research in the previous section has established that there is a close association between parental and child adjustment in all the conditions – cardiac disorders, diabetes and haemophilia – that are the concern of this review. Although the literature on these disorders contains considerable discussion on the emotional problems of the parents much is based on clinical impressions. Few studies have compared attitudes of the parents with those of parents of non-handicapped children or examined the extent of emotional problems in a representative sample of the parents.

Cardiac Disorders

Only a few studies are addressed specifically to the subject of family adjustment to a child with a cardiac handicap, and as with haemophilia and diabetes, mothers have been studied more often than the whole family. Only Maxwell and Gane (1962) have investigated parents' understanding of the handicap, their reaction on first hearing about it, and their attitudes to surgery, together with the effect on family life, problems of caring for the child, and effect on siblings. They found only 14 per cent of their sample of parents who were considered completely unable to adjust to the situation. However, at the time of the diagnosis nearly all reported having reacted with shock and concern. Some of the researchers suggest that an awareness of the vital role of the heart to life may mean that congenital heart disorder has a greater emotional impact than other serious disorders (Glaser *et al.*, 1964; Apley *et al.*, 1967; Landtman *et al.*, 1968 (see Section I)).

Over half of Maxwell and Gane's subjects stated that the care of the handicapped child gave rise to problems, and about a third felt that siblings were adversely affected. Some of the children, of course, have more obvious symptoms than others. Glaser *et al.*'s (1964) sample was smaller, but they also list many sources of stress and worry, in particular conflict about whether to restrict the child's activities, and anxiety about surgery. These were also findings of Boon's (1972) study in Newcastle. Mothers reported being restricted in their social lives and having to defer taking up work outside the home, and there were extra expenses to be met. Siblings often resented the handicapped child being 'spoiled', but parents were anxious to avoid cyanotic attacks. When parents of 260 children in Texas were interviewed by Garson *et al.* (1978) the same kinds of stress were disclosed once again: anxieties about symptoms, about what to tell the child, and about restriction of activity. Both Garson and Maxwell and Gane found parents, not surprisingly, unclear about the actual medical condition.

Delay in confirmation of the initial diagnosis had a disturbing emotional effect on parents (Glaser *et al.*, 1964; Apley *et al.*, 1967). Apley *et al.* found that more than half of the mothers in their sample, including a third of those judged to be well adjusted, were dissatisfied to some extent with diagnostic consultations at hospitals. Parental anxiety was partly responsible for poor communication but insufficient explanation and assurance by doctors added to the difficulties. Several studies recommend better support and explanation for the cardiac child's parents, but an experimental programme of extra support reported by Kupst *et al.* (1977) had inconclusive effects.

For most children with congenital heart defects the treatment is surgery. 83 per cent of the parents in Maxwell and Gane's study (1962) welcomed the prospect. Landtman *et al.* (1968) (see Section I) found that extreme maternal anxiety about the operation became less frequent over the period of their long-term study, during which cardiac operations became much more common. In Landtman's earlier (1960) study he reported that once the operation was over many mothers found it easier to relate to a child with greatly improved health. Nevertheless surgery involves stress for parents, the decision being particularly difficult if the child is without symptoms (Glaser *et al.*, 1964; Landtman *et al.*, 1968). It is clear that parents of children with cardiac defects have many common problems from the time the condition is first suspected.

Haemophilia

In the families of haemophiliacs, the mother's ability to cope with the situation is once again stressed as being vital to the child's adjustment and to the family atmosphere. Reports on the role of fathers are scarce and contradictory, Meijer (1980) finding that they took less part than most fathers in caring for the children, and Markova and Forbes (1979), Markova *et al.* (1980a) and Mattson and Gross (1966, see Section I) finding that they took a specially active part.

Mattson and Gross conclude that the 77 per cent of their group of haemophiliac boys who were well adjusted had mothers who could manage well in spite of their anxieties, while the remainder of the mothers had problems with over-protectiveness and pessimism. Madden *et al.* (1982) also found a strong relationship between the mother's acceptance of the illness and good adjustment in the child, and the former was helped along by support from the father and the rest of the family. Contrary to Meyers *et al.*'s (1972) conclusion that family stress was related to the severity of the illness, Madden *et al.* found no relation between the two.

Families with a haemophiliac child nevertheless have severe problems to surmount. A small group of New York parents investigated by Salk *et al.* (1972) reported social restrictions (nearly half the group) and financial strain (three-quarters). Nearly half reported a negative effect on their marriage, and 53 per cent had decided to have no more children. 82 per cent of the parents felt they had accepted the illness, though nearly all had found the diagnosis devastating at first. Meijer (1980) found mothers of haemophiliacs to be significantly more depressed than mothers of healthy children, and Madden *et al.* report severe anxiety about bleeding episodes. They found this to be more important than feelings of guilt about transmitting the disease, though Browne *et al.* (1960) and Mattson and Gross (1966) report guilt in the mothers of haemophiliacs even where there was no known family history of the disease.

A study carried out in Scotland (Markova and Forbes, 1979; Markova *et al.*, 1980a) suggests a more positive side to the haemophiliac's family. The authors found that, particularly where the handicap was not overwhelmingly severe, parents were providing a more carefully structured upbringing for the handicapped child than were parents of healthy children. Other studies (Mattson and Gross, 1966; Meijer, 1980; Meyers *et al.*, 1972) suggest difficulties, as with both the other handicaps reviewed here, in knowing how far to be protective and to restrict potentially dangerous activities. The problem is particularly acute for the parents of the haemophiliac. Parents may realize that haemophiliac boys need the same experiences as other children yet fear the consequences of accident. Research suggests, though, that haemophiliac children may come to set their own self-limits at an early age and can protect themselves against body contact injuries (Goldy and Katz, 1963 (see Section I)). The psychological consequences of over-protection appear to be more harmful than minor injuries (Goldy and Katz, 1963; Agle, 1964 (see Section I)). This is a point on which parents need guidance and reassurance from their doctors.

Diabetes

There is not very much research evidence about the families of diabetics. Two studies which explored problems of emotional adjustment in diabetic children did, however, also consider parental adjustment (Sterky, 1963; Swift *et al.*, 1967 (see Section I)). Sterky found a significantly higher proportion of mental disturbance in mothers of diabetic children living in Stockholm than in mothers of matched non-diabetic children; anxiety – possibly a quite realistic reaction – was the commonest symptom. Swift and his associates found more turmoil and conflict in the homes of New Jersey diabetic children than in those of controls. Mothers in Börner and Steinhausen's study (1977) assessed themselves as reserved, depressed, and lacking in self-confidence, and another study (Crain *et al.*, 1966b), particularly concerned with family functioning, found that parents of diabetic children in two areas of the United States had poorer marital relationships than those of non-diabetic children. In a study by Watson (1972) eight of the 15 parents interviewed were judged to have an 'unacceptably high' level of anxiety and distress. It is not impossible, if the psychosomatic view of diabetes is taken, that these findings are contributory to the child becoming diabetic rather than the result of it, or – more likely – that there is a complex interaction and feedback between all members of a family.

Watson also investigated the adequacy of services provided for the family with a diabetic. Parents reported that they had not been given enough explanation or a chance to discuss the illness, and were left to cope on their own from the start. Supportive home visits would have been very much welcomed. Although most of the parents coped with management after a time, nearly all were frightened about the possibility of hypoglycaemic or ketotic episodes and of the child becoming unconscious. Communication between hospital and the school authorities was equally poor. In general the understanding of the illness has not been found to be as good as it should be (Watson, 1972; Delbridge, 1975; Kronenfeld and Ory, 1981).

Investigators have also been interested in the question of daily management of the disease. Good management, not unexpectedly, has been found to be related to good family adjustment (Delbridge, 1975; Allen *et al.*, 1984). Allen and his associates investigated the child's responsibility for management and found adolescents to be more rebellious about their regime than younger children. In the small group studied by

Kronenfeld and Ory (1981), children and mothers had different perceptions of the difficulties of management, mothers being concerned with diet and children more with their injections and with restrictions on their social lives. These authors urge that, like haemophiliacs and cardiac children, diabetics should be restricted as little as is reasonably feasible.

The only study examining the complexity of family interaction as a whole is the ingenious procedure carried out by Baker and his associates (1975). In an attempt to find out why some diabetic children have frequent unexplained bouts of acidosis, an arrangement was made for repeated blood sampling and monitoring of free fatty acids; at the same time a family task was set that would demonstrate typical family interactions. There was found to be a definite correlation between the child's role in family conflict and a rise in free fatty acid levels leading to acidosis. The pressure of anxiety within the diabetic's family may be a two-way process.

Many of the problems faced by parents of diabetic children then appear very similar to the problems of haemophiliacs and children with cardiac handicaps. The close involvement of parents in the child's management, though, and the possibility of harmful effects if this is not carried out adequately, present unique features. They make it essential for parents of diabetic children to have the opportunity to discuss their fears and anxieties and to be given explanations which they fully understand.

MAXWELL, G.M. and GANE, S. (1962) *American Heart Journal*, 64, 4, 449–54.

The impact of congenital heart disease upon the family

150 families of children with congenital heart disease attending a clinic in Wisconsin were studied. Only 58 per cent had more than superficial knowledge of congenital heart disease, and misconceptions as to prognosis were common. Diagnosis had usually been made before the child was five years old by the family's private physician, and 'worry', 'fright' and 'concern' were reactions in 90 per cent of the parents. 75 per cent said they were satisfied with the initial consultation, but 40 per cent had sought other medical advice. 59 per cent thought that care of the child gave rise to problems – discipline (50 per cent) and feeding (20 per cent) being the most common. 32 per cent thought the child might suddenly die.

Most (60 per cent) thought the child's condition had not affected marital relationships. 38 per cent considered that the siblings were adversely affected, mainly by worry (18 per cent) or hostility and jealousy (10 per cent). 14 per cent of families were completely unable to 'adjust' to the situation and adjustment in some of the other families was tenuous. The majority (70 per cent) of parents reacted favourably to the possibility of surgery.

Measures by which a physician can help to alleviate some of these anxieties include: (1) presenting a definite diagnosis as soon as possible – and giving repeated simple explanations of this; (2) giving reassurance that the child will not suddenly die; (3) explaining that the parents are not to blame for the child's defect; (4) telling parents about the natural history of the disease so they can cope with problems as they arise, e.g. respiratory infections; (5) encouraging as much physical activity as the child's condition allows.

GLASER, H.H., HARRISON, G.S., and LYNN, D.B. (1964) *Pediatrics*, 33, 367–79.

Emotional implications of congenital heart disease in children

Twenty-five mothers of children with congenital heart defects (12 already operated on) were interviewed. Emotional strains on many of the mothers included: vague anxiety about the child before the diagnosis was made; lack of certainty about the child's condition even after the diagnosis; fear of sudden illness or death during the child's early years; difficulties in care of an infant with poor growth and irritable temperament; centring attention on the child at the expense of the rest of the family; self-blame for the child's condition; worry about the child's ability to lead a 'normal' life; fears about permitting the physical activities advised by doctors; uncertainty over discipline; conflict of feelings about accepting recommendation for surgery; concern about the child's own fearfulness of his or her condition; apprehension about cardiac catheterization, the operation itself and its outcome. If the family physician is aware of these problems he or she can do much to alleviate them.

CRAIN, A.J., SUSSMAN, M.B., and WEIL, W.B. Jr. (1966a) *International Journal of Social Psychiatry* 12, 35–43.

Family interaction, diabetes and sibling relationships

The social-psychological functioning of diabetic children (measured by self-esteem, satisfaction with behaviour, level of aspiration and academic achievement) was found not to differ significantly from that of siblings of diabetic children. In diabetic children it was closely related to the mother's behaviour, but there was no similar relationship between social-psychological functioning of the non-diabetic sibling and mother's behaviour. Subjects were 19 diabetic children aged 8 to 11 years attending a diabetes research clinic and 16 children of similar age who had diabetic siblings attending the same clinic.

CRAIN, A.J., SUSSMAN, M.B., and WEIL, W.B. Jr. (1966b) *Journal of Health and Human Behaviour,* 7, 2, 122–7.

Effects of a diabetic child on marital integration and related measures of family functioning

On standardized scales, parents of diabetic children had significantly poorer marital relationships, a tendency towards more marital conflicts, and greater disagreement over the children's actions than parents of non-diabetic children. Subjects were the middle and lower-middle class parents of 54 diabetic and 76 matched non-diabetic children. It can be argued that the lower marital integration of the parents of diabetics could have existed before the onset of the illness and could have been an aetiological factor – previous research has suggested that disrupting family circumstances may precipitate diabetes in children who are genetically predisposed to the illness. It is more likely, though, that the lower marital integration is the outcome of the continuous crisis situation in the family caused by the diabetes.

APLEY, J., BARBOUR, R.F., and WESTMACOTT, I. (1967) *British Medical Journal,* i, 103–5.

Impact of congenital heart disease on the family: preliminary report

In 88 families of children with congenital heart disease living in Bristol or the south-west, 39 per cent of mothers had been excessively disturbed by the initial shock of the diagnosis. Family balance was upset (e.g. father changed job, house reorganized) in 54 per cent of the families, and social activities were restricted in 36 per cent. Siblings showed behaviour problems in 27 per cent of families. Severity of the heart defect appeared to play some role in determining the impact on the family, disturbances in family life being much more common in families of the 12 children with incurable cardiac conditions than in those (not included in the series) who were declared free of defect after some years of hospital attendance.

Sixty mothers, judged to be 'specifically over-reacting' (over-protective or rejecting) were compared with 28 mothers judged to be well-adjusted. The 'specifically over-reacting' mothers were more likely to be generally immature, not satisfied with the interview, to have families in which the balance was upset, be prone to anxiety, to be excessively upset by the diagnosis, to have a restricted social life; they were less likely to leave the child with neighbours or let the sibling play normally with the child.

Delays and uncertainties in confirmation of the diagnosis and delay in the operation were associated with over-anxiety and disturbance in family patterns. 36 per cent of well-adjusted mothers as well as 75 per cent of the 'specifically over-reacting' mothers were not completely satisfied with the diagnostic consultation.

OFFORD, D.R. and APONTE, J.F. (1967) *Journal of the American Academy of Child Psychiatry*, 6, 3, 499.

Distortion of disability and effect on family life

Contrary to the expectations of the authors, children who had congenital heart disease with symptoms did not differ in personal adjustment from children with congenital heart disease but no symptoms (as evaluated by a psychiatrist from a battery of psychological tests and an interview); mothers of the children with symptoms were not more over-protective (measured by restrictions not advised by the physician which were placed on the child); nor was the family life of this group more affected by the disorder.

The mother's perception of the illness was the key factor in its effect on family life. Mothers who overestimated the severity of the child's defect (compared with the cardiologist's rating) had the highest over-protection scores, followed by mothers who underestimated the severity, while over-protection was least for those who saw the child's defect accurately; families of the overestimating mothers were also the most affected by the heart defect and those of mothers with accurate perceptions were least affected. No significant differences were found, though, between child adjustment in the three groups. Mothers who had lived longest with the illness were most likely to overrate its severity. Subjects were 19 children, aged 4 to 15 years, admitted to the

University of Florida Teaching Hospital for cardiac evaluation, and their mothers.

BOON, A.R.
(1972)
British Journal of Preventive and Social Medicine,
26, 4, 263–9.

Tetralogy of Fallot – effect on the family

One hundred patients in Newcastle were studied, ranging from a few months old to 28 years. The families were visited to ascertain what their problems had been; 47 normal families with a child of the same age were used as a comparison for parts of the study. It was found that parents had to go through a great deal of strain in coping with the condition, as well as having extra expenses. Mothers of the affected children reported more restrictions on their own recreation than mothers in the control group. Work outside the home was usually deferred for them until the cardiac child was at school or had had surgery. The effect on having further children was not great, though there was a tendency for the next birth to be postponed for a time. After corrective surgery nearly all the children were able to go to normal schools, they lost less time with respiratory infections, and they became more active and healthy. Out of 46 operations carried out within the group, however, there had been seven deaths.

MEYERS, R.D. *et al.*
(1972)
American Journal of Public Health,
62, 530–5.

The social and economic impact of haemophilia – a survey of 70 cases in Vermont and New Hampshire

A study of all the haemophiliacs who could be located in Vermont and New Hampshire. A correlation was found between the severity of the disorder and family stress, but strains sometimes occurred even where the illness was mild. Understanding of the illness alleviated tensions in the families of mild haemophiliacs but could not prevent fears in the families of the severely affected. Conflict over sports activities was common between parents and the haemophiliac children, particularly where the child was severely affected. Lack of advice from their physician often resulted in parents being unnecessarily restrictive. Only six of the haemophiliacs who were of school age or over were not receiving or had not received their education within the public school system. Schools, though, like parents, tended to place unnecessary restrictions on the child. Only one haemophiliac in the sample had received vocational guidance. 55 per cent of the adult haemophiliacs had experienced some difficulty in their present employment because of their illness. Improvements in vocational guidance, family planning advice and cover of medical expenses are necessary if the problems of the haemophiliac are to be eased.

OFFORD, D.R., CROSS, L.A., ANDREWS, E.J., and APONTE, J.F. (1972) *Psychosomatics*, 13, 390–6.

Perceived and actual severity of congenital heart disease and effect on family life

Subjects were 20 children aged 9 to 17 with suspected or confirmed heart disease, seen at a hospital in Florida. Mothers' ages ranged from 30 to 48, and their educational level ranged from a few years' schooling to postgraduate status. Children and mothers were interviewed separately, and children's interviewers knew nothing about the children's background. From the interviews with mothers, an effect-on-family-life score was compiled from questions about family arrangements and about over-protection of the child. The children themselves were asked about work, play, friends, and future plans. The cardiologist also recorded his opinion of the child's health status, making three independent views altogether of the severity of the illness. When results were compared, it was clear that the mother's view of the severity of the disease was more important than its actual severity in influencing the effect on the child and on family life. The mothers from the poorer families were more likely to misunderstand the nature of the disease. (See also Offord and Aponte, 1967.)

SALK, L., HILGARTNER, M., and GRANICH, B. (1972) *Social Science and Medicine*, 6, 491–505.

The psycho-social impact of hemophilia on the patient and his family

Twenty-six children attending a New York clinic and their parents were interviewed. The sample was mainly white and middle-class. Only 31 per cent had a known family history of haemophilia. The impact of learning of the disease was said to have been devastating by most of the parents, though 83 per cent felt they had now accepted it. Nearly half reported that it had had a negative effect on their marriage (most of the children, however, felt that the illness had no bad effects on the family). 43 per cent of the families felt socially restricted, and 75 per cent reported financial strain. 53 per cent had decided not to have more children.

Of the children, 63 per cent were considered by their parents to have adjusted to haemophilia, and about the same number reported themselves that this was so. 19 per cent of the children said they felt resentful or afraid. While 69 per cent said their physical lives were limited, only 15 per cent said that friendships were. 83 per cent had had spontaneous bleedings; there was a distinct peak between February and May, and a peak on Tuesdays, the day of the clinic. More guidance for parents is recommended.

WATSON, A. (1972) *Community Medicine,* 128, 5, 122–5.

A study of family attitudes to children with diabetes

Fifteen families randomly selected from all families with diabetic children in two London boroughs were interviewed in their homes. Initial reactions were shock at the diagnosis followed by anxiety about diabetic management. Parents felt that they had no opportunity to discuss their feelings about the diagnosis. Teaching of parents at the eight hospitals attended by the children was only barely or less than adequate. Few parents received home visits from any professional worker in the first few weeks although these would have been welcomed. By the time of the interview 11 families could cope with management techniques. Nevertheless the interviewer considered that eight of the 15 parents had an unacceptably high level of anxiety and stress; distress was related to inadequate understanding of diabetes and lack of confidence in being able to control it, both of which were found mainly in lower social class parents.

From interviews with schools it was found that there was little anxiety about having a diabetic pupil but also little knowledge of the illness and its management, although dietary needs were understood. Parents turned to the hospital for advice about diabetes, but hospitals were generally only concerned with the child's medical condition and not his or her social situation. Communication between hospitals and local authorities (at present rare) suggesting advice and support for some families, and between the hospitals and the schools (at present non-existent) to give them initial information, would help to solve some of the problems.

BAKER, L., MINUCHIN, S., MILMAN, S., LIEBMAN, R., and TODD, T. (1975) *Modern Problems in Pediatrics,* 12, 332–43.

Psychosomatic aspects of juvenile diabetes mellitus: a progress report

An attempt was made to determine whether diabetic children who have multiple bouts of acidosis for which there is no organic explanation are in fact reacting psychosomatically to stresses within the family. Individual children were admitted to a clinical research centre in Pennsylvania. Long-acting insulin was withdrawn and the child maintained on doses of short-acting insulin. A small needle was inserted in a peripheral vein with a stopcock arrangement that allowed for frequent blood sampling. The child's family was assembled and a family task set, which was then video-taped; a detailed family diagnostic interview was also carried out. During this time free fatty acids in the diabetic's blood, representing emotional arousal leading to acidosis, was frequently monitored. There was a definite correlation between the child's role in family conflict and free fatty acid levels. A beta adrenergic blocking agent was also administered to the child in order to lower arousal. Of six children studied in this way, three showed moderate improvement and one had a complete cessation of unexplained ketoacidosis.

DELBRIDGE, L. (1975) *The Medical Journal of Australia,* 2, 737–9.

Educational and psychological factors in the management of diabetes in childhood

Management of diabetes, attitudes towards it, and family adjustment were studied in a group of 37 diabetic children and their parents in Australia. Good understanding and acceptance of the illness was related to good management of it and to good family adjustment. Overall the children showed inadequate understanding of their illness and rather poor social adjustment.

KOSKI, M.-L., AHLAS, A., and KUMENTO, A. (1976) *Acta Paedopsychiatrica,* 42, 12–26.

A psychosomatic follow-up study of childhood diabetes

Follow-up of an earlier study; 53 children and young people in Finland were re-examined to determine their progress. As well as physical examinations, semistructured psychiatric interviews were held with each subject, and diabetic control was also assessed. Where subjects had changed from good to poor control (11 cases), tragedies such as parental death, divorce, or illness had occurred. Where they had changed from poor to good control (nine cases), better medical care was involved, or the resolution of a depression. Good diabetic control was strongly associated with healthy family functioning. Thirty-four out of the 53 children were average or above average in school achievement.

BÖRNER, S. and STEINHAUSEN, H.C. (1977) *Pediatric and Adolescent Endocrinology,* 3, 46–51.

A psychological study of family characteristics in juvenile diabetes

An assessment of the personalities of 76 parents of diabetics, together with 13 adolescent diabetics. Parents and children both filled in standardized self-report questionnaires. The resulting personality profiles suggested that mothers of diabetics tend to be reserved, depressed, and lacking in self-confidence, while fathers presented a similar profile to fathers of healthy children. There was no difference in personality patterns between mothers of children with good diabetic control and poor control. The group of adolescents saw themselves as having more negativity than parents saw in them, which suggests that parents do not reinforce any feelings the adolescent has of being stigmatized.

KUPST, M.J., BLATTERBAUER, S., WESTMAN, J., SCHULMAN, J.L., and PAUL, M.H. (1977) *Pediatrics*, 59, 2, 266–72.

Helping parents cope with the diagnosis of congenital heart defect: an experimental study

Parents often find it difficult to understand the implications of their child's congenital heart defect. In this study a social worker was used to help parents understand, guide them towards coping effectively, and allow emotions to surface. Subjects were 84 parents attending a cardiac out-patient clinic for the first time in Chicago assigned to four groups of 21: those simply given a fuller explanation of the diagnosis by the social worker (medical information only), those encouraged to discuss problems with her (psychological), those combining both these approaches (medical-psychological), and a control group who were only seen by the doctor. Ratings of anxiety and of parent satisfaction were made, and all parents were tested right afterwards and one month later on their understanding of the heart condition. The average recall of the three groups who had had extra discussion was higher than that of the controls, but a month later there were no significant differences. There were no differences in anxiety level or satisfaction with the visit.

GARSON, A., SCOTT BENSON, R., IVLER, L., and PATTON, C. (1978) *Child Psychiatry and Human Development*, 9, 86–94.

Parental reactions to children with congenital heart disease

Unstructured interviews were held with the parents of 260 children attending a cardiology clinic in Texas. A number of questions which they found it difficult to ask emerged: 'Was I responsible for the defect?' 'Why did it take so long to diagnose?' 'What exactly is the defect?' 'What symptoms should we look for?' 'What should we tell the child?' 'How far should we treat him normally?' Parents of children with different types of condition – pre- and post-operative, symptomatic and asymptomatic – reacted differently for each of these conditions. Parents need emotional support, especially those with less severely ill children who receive less attention from clinic staff.

MARKOVA, I. and FORBES, C. (1979) *Health Bulletin*, 37, 1, 24–9.

Haemophilia: a study into social and psychological problems

A small group of haemophiliacs and their parents in Scotland were studied. Sixteen parents of haemophiliacs were interviewed and compared with eight control parents. In the former group, fathers had helped more with the children during infancy. The haemophiliac children had been given more rules and responsibilities than children in control families, though this was less true of the severely affected. Mothers in the haemophiliac group worried more about their children's futures than control mothers. Half of the mothers of haemophiliacs had affected relatives, but only three of these had thought they might be carriers; about half of those who did not think of being carriers wished they had known in advance. Interviews were also given to eight haemophiliac schoolboys; though none were very positive about their schools, those at residential schools were more dissatisfied. None were very realistic about future careers.

MARKOVA, I., MACDONALD, K. and FORBES, C. (1980a) *Journal of Child Psychology and Psychiatry,* 21, 2, 153–62.

Impact of haemophilia on child-rearing practices and parental co-operation

Another account of part of the research reported in Markova and Forbes (1979). The family dynamics where there is a haemophiliac child are discussed, in particular the fact that where the handicap is mild the parents seem to be stimulated to provide a particularly well-structured upbringing. Knowledge of the family history is discussed, and genetic counselling.

MEIJER, A. (1980) *International Journal of Psychiatry in Medicine,* 10, 2, 163–72.

Psychiatric problems of hemophilic boys and their families

Special emotional risks within the haemophiliac's family have been described: guilt and resentment in parents, anxiety and dependence, or else risk-taking behaviour, in the child. The aim of the study was to examine these problems. Four questionnaires were administered to 20 mothers of haemophiliacs and 20 control mothers, all living in Israel. The former were found to have significantly more depressed feelings. There was a trend for fathers of haemophiliacs to be seen as less involved with their sons than the fathers of healthy children were. The haemophiliac children were seen as defiant by their mothers, which is contrasted with the author's previous findings on compliant behaviour in asthmatic children. The defiance is likely to be a reaction against anxiety and dependence.

ANDERSON, B.J., MILLER, J.P., AUSLANDER, W.F., and SANTIAGO, J.V. (1981) *Diabetes Care,* 4, 6, 586–94.

Family characteristics of diabetic adolescents: relationship to metabolic control

The family environments of 58 diabetic adolescents in Washington who were in good, fair, and poor control of the illness were compared. The families were 83 per cent Caucasian, 15 per cent black, and 2 per cent Hispanic, and were mainly of a middle to upper middle-class level. Structured interviews were held with young people and with parents, and the young people completed standard scales assessing self-concept and family environment.

25 per cent of the sample were considered to be in good control, 54 per cent fair, and 21 per cent poor, and there was no relation to class, family size, or age. Those in poor control reported more symptoms such as visual problems and fatigue. On the self-concept scale, average scores were higher than the norm. Well-controlled adolescents scored significantly higher than the others, while the poorly controlled group scored significantly on anxiety. The well-controlled group also reported more cohesion and less conflict within the family. More of the parents of well-controlled young people stated that family members were encouraged to be independent. In addition, more parents of the poorly controlled group stated that diabetes had negatively affected the young person's personality, well-being, and schooling. These findings suggest a complex interplay between the adolescents' psychological and physical functioning, metabolic control, and the family environment.

KRONENFELD, J.K. and ORY, M.G. (1981) *Postgraduate Medicine,* 70, 4, 83–90.

Familial perceptions of juvenile diabetes

Ten diabetic children and their mothers, from a hospital clinic in Alabama, were interviewed about their main concerns and dislikes in living with diabetes. Half the children were from white households and half from black, and the families were mostly working-class. Children and mothers had rather different perceptions of the difficulties, mothers focusing on diet, and children on the dislike of injections and on social restrictions. None of the children expressed a fear that diabetes might affect any future plans to marry, but both mothers and children expressed anxiety about future job possibilities. Mothers seemed to be over-cautious in restricting the children's social activities. It is suggested that doctors should give as accurate information as possible to families, and in particular make sure that diabetic children are not restricted too much.

KLEIN, R.H. and NIMORWICZ, P. (1982) *Journal of Psychosomatic Research,* 26, 4, 387–91.

The relationship between psychological distress and knowledge of disease among hemophiliac patients and their families: a pilot study

As part of a larger scale study, 12 pilot families were assessed for knowledge of haemophilia and for depression and anxiety. Mothers reported most signs of distress, followed by adolescent children; fathers reported least distress and children under 15 little or none. Mothers scored 75 per cent correct on knowledge of the illness, under-fifteens 69 per cent, fathers 67 per cent, and over-fifteens 65 per cent.

MADDEN, N.A., TERRIZZI, J., and FRIEDMAN, S.B. (1982) *Journal of Developmental and Behavioral Pediatrics,* 3, 3, 136–42.

Psychological issues in mothers of children with hemophilia

Twenty-four mothers of haemophiliac sons took part in semi-structured interviews, which were converted to 5-point scales of Child Adjustment and of Maternal Psychological Response to Haemophilia. Ratings were also made for guilt, fearfulness, and family support. Family support was found to be associated with acceptance of the illness. Few mothers expressed strong guilt, and fearfulness about bleeding episodes was more prominent. A strong relationship was found between mother's acceptance of haemophilia and good adjustment in the child. None was found between severity of illness and maladjustment, nor between severity of illness and mothers' acceptance of it. The limitations of a self-reporting method are stressed, but also that guidance and support emerge as extremely important.

ALLEN, A.A., TENNEN, H., MCGRADE, B.J., AFFLECK, G., and RATZAN, S. (1984) *Journal of Pediatric Psychology,* 8, 2, 129–41.

Parent and child perceptions of the management of juvenile diabetes

Subjects were 34 children aged 8 to 17 from a diabetic clinic in Connecticut. Interviews with each child and parent were conducted simultaneously in different rooms; they were asked to rate the extent to which the child took responsibility for several aspects of management, whether this was considered satisfactory, and how much they minded the restrictions. For each one, clinic staff made ratings of compliance and of coping. Metabolic control was assessed from medical records. Parents and children did not differ in their accounts of management responsibility, and no child or parent reported that the child had too much responsibility. Parents who allowed their children to take responsibility for diet tended to be those who were rated as coping well. Children in poorer control were more likely to be giving themselves their own insulin injections; average age of those who sometimes, usually, and always took this responsibility was 10.8, 12, and 12.3 years. Adolescents were rated as having poorer compliance than younger children. Children with early onset of the illness took more responsibility than those with late onset. In general, parents' views of metabolic control differed from those of the professionals.

SECTION III

Educational Attainments

There is very little research on the educational attainments of children with physical disorders not involving the brain. A recent study has been made, though, which compares the intelligence and educational attainments of all 10- to 12-year-old children with physical disorders living on the Isle of Wight with those of the general population (Yule and Rutter, 1970). The children with physical disorders (excluding those with asthma and eczema) were found, on average, to be slightly below the control group in intelligence. Significantly more of the children with physical disorders (16.67 per cent) than of the general population (5.4 per cent) were reading at a level 28 months or more below that expected for their age and intelligence. At least part of the explanation for this educational retardation was found in the high rate of absence from school of the children with physical disorders. Again, of course, these findings do not necessarily apply to all the disorders under review and it is useful to consider the available research for each condition separately.

Cardiac Disorders

Although there is no research specifically on cardiac children's school achievement, a good deal of interest has been shown in the effects of a heart defect, and of a heart operation, on intelligence; but as a result of the range of impairment that may be shown by the child in this mixed group the results are complex. Where overall intelligence level is concerned, groups of children with cardiac handicaps have been found to fall within the average limits for their age (Drash and Money, 1968; Honzik *et al.,* 1969; Bayer, 1976; O'Dougherty *et al.,* 1983). When sub-groups and specific types of ability are examined in more detail, however, there appear to be some differences from group to group.

A number of studies have been concerned with the effect of cyanosis. Children with cyanotic heart defects have lowered blood-oxygen levels and there is a possibility that this may have a damaging effect on intelligence. In all available studies which examine cyanotic and acyanotic children separately, the cyanotic children have lower average intelligence, although still within the normal range (Linde *et al.,* 1966 (see Section I); Rasof *et al.,* 1967; Feldt *et al.,* 1969; Silbert *et al.,* 1969).

It is not yet clear why cyanotic children have lower intelligence. While it remains possible that the lowered arterial oxygen saturation is the primary factor, findings of the studies carried out by Linde, Rasof, and their associates (Linde *et al.*, 1966; Rasof *et al.*, 1967) suggest that the associated physical incapacity may be of greater importance, as it interferes with the child's early manipulative experiences. The relationship found between incapacity and intelligence in young children tended to disappear in older children. The intelligence of the older cyanotic children was significantly higher than that of the younger ones. It appears from this study that cyanotic children are able to catch up on experiences after they learn to walk and are also able to perform better on the measures of intelligence used for older groups, which emphasize verbal abilities, rather than those used in the early years, which rely mainly on sensory-motor functions.

An alternative explanation is suggested by Feldt *et al.* (1969), who did not find higher scores in the older children. They noted an association between small head circumference, growth failure, and low intelligence. The authors suggest that an adverse pre-natal factor might simultaneously affect the heart, brain, and other tissues of the developing foetus, or that infant malnutrition, connected with the cardiac defect, results in deficiencies in brain development. Differences in the samples of children studied may be relevant to these opposed points of view. Silbert *et al.* (1969) also found growth retardation in a small group of cyanotic children as opposed to acyanotic ones, together with late development, incapacity for strenuous play, and rather poorer scores on tests of visual perception and motor performance than those of acyanotic or normal children. The authors link cyanosis with impaired central nervous system function.

In general the IQ of children with congenital heart defects has been found to be higher after operation than before (Drash and Money, 1968; Landtman *et al.*, 1968 (see Section I); Linde *et al.*, 1970 (see Section I)), but with several qualifications. O'Dougherty *et al.* (1983) found earlier surgery to be associated with better intelligence scores. Bayer and Honzik (1976) and Honzik *et al.* (1976) followed up 334 children for some years and concluded that reports of the pathogenic effect of cardiac illness and cardiac operation were unfounded. Both intelligence and adjustment were average. But on a test of perceptual-motor ability the children were below average both before and after surgery. The authors suggest that in spite of average intelligence there may have been some deficit. There could be support for the idea in O'Dougherty *et al.*'s finding, in a study of children who had undergone surgery for transposition of the great arteries, that in spite of an overall average intelligence level there were a number of abnormal neurological findings and abnormal EEG records. O'Dougherty and his associates, unlike most authors, also investigated the effect of social class and family stress, and found lower scores on intelligence, behaviour, and growth to be associated with lower social class and more stress.

O'Dougherty *et al.* also found a wider spread of intelligence in their sample, which contained both more gifted children and more retarded children than would be expected. Another factor in intelligence distribution was noted by Honzik and associates (1969, 1976): girls, who normally have higher verbal sub-scores than boys, consistently scored lower than boys on this sub-test in their investigations. So although the intelligence of children with cardiac handicaps has been found to fall within the normal range, findings are affected by cyanosis, by variation on sub-tests, by possible neurological involvement, and by sex and class.

Finally, there has been research isolating the effect of the use of deep hypothermia and circulatory arrest during major heart surgery on children. This is a matter for detailed medical appraisal, but it can be said that studies suggest that where subsequent lags in development or maturation have been found, they seem more likely to have been due to the effect of cyanosis or to pre-existing defects.

Haemophilia

Where haemophiliac children are concerned, research emphasis has been on school achievement, particularly on ascertaining the level that can be reached in spite of being handicapped by frequent absences with bleeding episodes. Most of the research inevitably dates back in time somewhat, especially where it is a question of young adults being quizzed about childhood experiences; it may not be representative of conditions obtaining today.

The two most ambitious projects are those of Katz (1970) in the USA and the Haemophilia Society (1977) in Britain, covering 1055 and 750 subjects respectively. Katz found that (in the 1950s and 60s) 34 per cent of haemophiliac boys in the United States did not complete high school and only 12 per cent graduated from a university. It was pointed out both by teachers and the boys' families that their illness prevented them from reaching the academic level they would ordinarily have done, and there was a higher rate of unemployment among the adults than in the general population. In Britain, the Haemophilia Society (1977) report that far fewer haemophiliacs than formerly are receiving inadequate education, and more are going on to higher education. Nevertheless the great majority who responded to their questionnaires stated that haemophilia had hindered their prospects, and over half of the employed adult subjects said they would not have chosen their current job if they had not been disabled.

That absence from school is the main problem is confirmed by Olch (1971b), who also found haemophiliacs performing below their age level, and missing on average twice as much schooling as the average child. In this American study home tutoring was considered inadequate and not enough supplementary help said to be given by teachers.

The same themes are taken up by two further British studies. Bronks and Blackburn (1968), unlike Katz in the USA, found that school leaving age of haemophiliacs in Britain compared favourably with that in the general population; nevertheless only 77 per cent of those who had left school were working. In Glasgow, Markova and her associates (1977, 1980b) found much that was unsatisfactory about haemophiliac boys' schooling. Time was constantly being lost through absence, with the sequel of poor qualifications and unsatisfying jobs. Home tuition was patchy and only provided during long absences. The authors stress in particular that teachers were not well informed and hospitals not putting out adequate communication. It is clear that educational services to fill this gap could be improved to the long-term benefit of haemophiliac children.

Only Olch has studied the actual intelligence profile of young haemophiliacs, as opposed to school attainment. He found that his sample fell within the high average range. Intellectual strengths and weaknesses were related to personal experience; the children were good with facts and with the manipulation of objects, probably because of spending time making models, reading, and watching television, but were relatively weak in areas needing understanding of social situations.

Diabetes

Where diabetes is concerned, all the research interest has gone into examination of psychosomatic aspects and emotional factors, rather than intelligence or school achievement. Since diabetics neither have such frequent absences from school as haemophiliac children, nor have to contend with major surgery like those with cardiac defects, one might expect their intelligence level to be average. This is, in fact, confirmed by several studies (Ack *et al.,* 1961; Weil and Ack, 1964; Fällström, 1974 (see Section I); Ludvigsson, 1977; Ahnsjö *et al.,* 1981).

There is some conflict, however, about educational achievement. Sterky (1963) in Sweden (see Section I), and Weil and Ack (1964), in Ohio, found their samples to be average performers in reading and arithmetic, while Gath *et al.* (1980), also in the United States, found reading backwardness to be significantly more common than in controls. The backwardness was related to poor family background and poor metabolic control. The two American studies do agree that age and onset of illness did not affect intelligence.

Fällström (1974) in fact found his group of diabetic children to be of *above* average intelligence. Some of the children had perceptual disturbances, however, which were associated with hypoglycaemic convulsions, abnormal EEG records, frequent hospitalizations, and low birthweight. But this was perhaps an unusual sample, as nearly a quarter had had perinatal complications. In Ack *et al.*'s (1961) sample, the few children who were under five had a lower average IQ than their control children; this lowered intelligence was related to episodes of hypoglycaemia and acidosis. Possibly these stresses caused temporary backwardness in younger children.

ACK, M., MILLER, I., and WEIL, W.B. Jr. (1961) *Pediatrics,* 28, 764–70.

Intelligence of child with diabetes mellitus

Thirty-eight diabetic children, attending the University Hospitals of Cleveland, were found to be similar in intelligence to their non-diabetic siblings; the 13 children who were under five years of age, though, were lower in intelligence than their controls. There was a tendency for episodes of hypoglycaemia and acidosis to be negatively related to intelligence in children under the age of five, but there was no relationship after this age. It is possible that these metabolic disturbances cause mental impairment in a young child but not in an older child. Alternatively, the stress of diabetes on the young child may cause the intellectual loss.

WEIL, W.B. Jr. and ACK, M. (1964) *Diabetes,* 13, 3, 303–6.

School achivement in juvenile diabetes mellitus

A further study of the diabetic children found in a previous investigation (Ack *et al.,* 1961) to be similar in intelligence to their non-diabetic siblings. Reading and arithmetic achievements of the diabetic children were those expected for their mental age. Performance, in relation to mental age, was similar for the diabetic children and their healthy siblings. Age of onset of diabetes was not related to academic achievements.

SOULIER, J.P. and JOSSO, F. (Eds) (1966) Basel, S. Karger, II Medico-Social Session, 2. 'The hemophiliac at school', 162–91.

Current Studies in Hemophilia. Proceedings of the 3rd Congress of the World Federation of Hemophilia, Paris, 1965.

Five papers, one by an English author and the others by French authors, discuss the medical and psychological problems of the haemophiliac boy at school. A possible solution is the specialized boarding school for haemophiliacs. One paper, by Dr Favre-Gilly and his associates, describes a school of this type which has been established in France for seven years.

RASOF, B., LINDE, L.M., and DUNN, O.J. (1967) *Child Development,* 38, 4, 1043–53.

Intellectual development in children with congenital heart disease

The question of whether intellectual functioning is adversely affected in children with cyanotic heart disease has been of concern to physicians and parents for a long time. In this study 98 children with cyanotic congenital heart disease were found to score significantly lower in intelligence than three other groups of children – 100 children with congenital heart disease but no cyanosis, 81 healthy siblings of the cardiac children and 40 normal children. The average IQ of the cyanotic children was within the normal range at every age level, however, and some had very high scores. Cyanotic children showed developmental delays in walking and speaking phrases compared with the acyanotic and normal children; however, the differences in intellectual level between the groups could not be accounted for by differences in factors such as age, sex, socio-economic level, or maternal attitudes.

In younger cardiac children a relationship was found between the level of incapacity and intelligence, but it tended to disappear in the older cardiac children. It is possible that the delay in mental development of the younger children is due to the defect itself, to the lowered arterial oxygen saturation, but it is more likely that the associated physical incapacity is the factor of primary importance. The relationship between incapacity and intelligence probably exists in the younger group because tests for this age range rely heavily on sensory-motor functions – and the child's physical incapacity limits manipulative experience and energy. The relationship tends to disappear in older children both because tests for this group emphasize verbal abilities and because the cardiac child tends to make up on early experience after he or she begins to walk. (See also Linde *et al.*, 1970 (Section I).)

BRONKS, I.G. and BLACKBURN, E.K. (1968) *British Journal of Preventive and Social Medicine*, 22, 68–72.

A socio-medical study of haemophilia and related states

A questionnaire survey carried out in 1964 of 135 patients with haemophilia or related disorders who had been referred to the Sheffield Royal Infirmary in the previous ten years. Forty-four were classified as being mildly affected, 21 as moderately affected, and 70 as severely affected. 57.1 per cent of those aged over 11 had attended secondary modern schools and 17.1 per cent grammar schools; only 11 attended special school and only three children did not go to school at all after the age of 11. School leaving age compared favourably with that of the general population.

77 per cent of the 87 subjects who had left school were working. 65 per cent of those who were severely affected were employed; only in this group were there any (42.5 per cent) who had been at work for less than 60 per cent of the time in the previous five years. 49.4 per cent of the subjects were married (significantly lower than for the general population) – there were no significant differences between the proportions of those married in the different grades of severity. The percentages of those in employment and married were very similar to those found by Katz, 1963 (see Section I). Only four subjects were living alone.

Nine subjects (6.7 per cent) stated that they had seen a psychiatrist, although only six had actually received psychiatric treatment. These figures appear to be comparable to those in the general population, suggesting that haemophilia does not cause overt psychiatric illness. Evidence on whether bleeding can be induced by emotional stress was inconclusive.

DRASH, P.W. and MONEY, J. (1968) In: D.B. CHEECK (Ed) *Human Growth. Body Composition, Cell Growth, Energy and Intelligence.* Philadelphia: Lea and Febiger, 606–15.

Statural and intellectual growth in congenital heart disease, in growth hormone deficiency and in sibling controls

The intelligence distributions of 20 children with unoperated congenital heart disorders and of ten children with congenital heart disorders who had undergone surgery were very close to the expected normal distribution. The mean IQ, though, of the post-operative group was slightly higher than that of the pre-operative group. Two of four children who had undergone open-heart surgery decreased considerably in performance IQ after the operation. The mean IQ of the cardiac group as a whole was 7.59 IQ points lower than that of their normal siblings. The unoperated cardiac children were slightly below average in height and there was a significant degree of correlation between height and intelligence in this group. The low intelligence was as likely to have been the consequence of the general low socio-economic status of this group or an artifact of sampling as to be connected with the growth retardation. No correlation between height and intelligence was found in a group of hypopituitary dwarfs with severe growth retardation.

FELDT, R.H., EWART, J.C., STICKLER, G.B., and WEIDMAN, W.H. (1969) *American Journal of Diseases of Children,* 117, 3, 281–7.

Children with congenital heart disease. Motor development and intelligence

Investigating intellectual retardation in children with congenital heart disease, the authors tested the intelligence of 78 subjects aged 2 to 17. Children with conditions affecting mental development, such as mongolism, were excluded. 9 per cent of the acyanotic children and 44 per cent of the cyanotic ones had IQs below 90. Ten children had a small head circumference; all were intellectually retarded. Another ten showed growth failure; six of these were retarded, four also having a small head circumference. No relation was found between severity of the cardiac defect or environmental deprivation and intelligence scores. The intelligence of 333 further children was assessed clinically and a similar relationship was found between intellectual retardation, small head circumference, and growth failure. Out of the whole sample, 226 children had head circumference measured and 14 per cent of these had a small circumference, less than would be expected in the general population, and all but one were retarded. These findings could be due to a teratogenic effect on heart and brain in the foetus or to infant malnutrition resulting in failure of normal brain development.

HONZIK, M.P., COLLART, D.S., ROBINSON, S.J., and FINLEY, K.H. (1969) *Science,* 164, 3878, 445–7.

Sex differences in verbal and performance IQs of children undergoing open-heart surgery

In normal samples no significant differences are found between the mental abilities of boys and girls, though girls do tend to be superior on tests of verbal ability while boys are superior on arithmetic tests and tests of spatial reasoning. Sixty boys and 58 girls aged 5 to 16 were tested six months after open-heart surgery, and contrary to the usual findings the girls tended to have significantly poorer scores on the verbal subscale than the boys. For boys the mean verbal IQ (104.2) did not differ significantly from the mean performance IQ (105.2). In contrast, the mean verbal IQ (95.8) of the girls was significantly lower than their mean performance IQ (99.5). Comparisons of the pre-operative sample and an enlarged post-operative sample with the normal distribution of IQ showed that the boys' verbal IQ distributions closely approximated the normal curve while the girls' verbal IQ distributions were both clearly below normal. The explanation may be environmental or a sex-associated genetic factor could be the cause.

SILBERT, A., WOLFF, P.H., MAYER, B., ROSENTHAL, A., and NADAS, A.S. (1969) *Pediatrics,* 43, 2, 192–200.

Cyanotic heart disease and psychological development

Three groups of children aged four to eight were studied, making 42 in all: one group with cyanotic heart disease, one with non-cyanotic heart disease who had experienced repeated episodes of congestive heart failure in infancy, and one with non-cyanotic heart disease who had never had congestive heart failure and were not discernibly handicapped. None of the children had other serious defects. The aim was to isolate the effect of cyanosis. A battery of tests of intelligence, perception, and coordination was administered, and parents were interviewed.

The cyanotic children scored significantly lower on the Binet intelligence test (averaging 105), some tests of visual perception, and tests of motor performance than children in the other two groups, the best scores being obtained by group 3. The cyanotic children also engaged in less vigorous activities, had developed later, and were more undersized than the others. Thus there appeared to be a direct relation between cyanosis due to congenital heart disease and impaired central nervous system function.

KATZ, A.H. (1970b) Springfield, Illinois: Charles C. Thomas. (Especially, Chapter 6, 'The education of hemophiliacs'; Chapter 7, 'Making a living'; and Chapter 8, 'Some special conditions: hemophilia and work', 39–88.)

Hemophilia. A Study in Hope and Reality

In a study of 1055 haemophiliacs over the age of 16 in the USA (see also Goldy and Katz, 1963; Katz, 1963 (Section I)) it was found that 65 per cent of the sample had been educated at ordinary schools and 14 per cent had received ordinary schooling as well as special schooling or home tuition; 64 per cent were or had been attending high school but 34 per cent did not complete it; 23 per cent received education beyond high school level, 12 per cent graduating from college. From discussions with haemophiliacs and their families and with school teachers it appeared that the academic achievements of the haemophiliac boy are generally below those expected for age and intelligence. To improve the quality of education for haemophiliacs, teachers need to acquire a greater understanding of haemophilia, so that fears and misconceptions are allayed and the child can be accepted in an ordinary class; provision of tuition during absences from school, whether in hospital or at home, is also needed.

82 per cent of the haemophiliacs in the survey were currently employed or still at school. There was a far higher rate of unemployment, though, than among the general population. 23 per cent were in professional or managerial jobs or owned their own businesses, 18 per cent were labourers and 54 per cent were in white collar or similar occupations. No real relationship was found between the severity of the illness and kind of occupation. Income for the employed tended to be higher than in the general population.

A comparison was made between the characteristics of the 'unsuccessful' (unemployed seven months or more)(105) and the 'successful' (employed)(447). The illness was more often of low severity in the 'successful' (in 50 per cent) than in the 'unsuccessful' (25 per cent). Subjects in the small group who were 'unsuccessful' although their illness was of low severity tended to emphasize their physical disability and to have 'given up', many having left school at an early age. Those who were 'unsuccessful' but whose illness was of high severity had to face real problems, but they probably tended to take a more negative attitude to themselves than did the 'successful'. The 'successful' subjects whose illness was of high severity (70) had tried to de-emphasize their handicap and aimed at living a normal life.

YULE, W. and RUTTER, M. (1970) In: RUTTER, M., TIZARD, J. and WHITMORE, K. (Eds) *Education, Health and Behaviour.* London: Longman, 297–308.

Educational aspects of physical disorder

The intelligence of 10- to 12-year-old children with physical disorders not involving the brain (orthopaedic disabilities, heart disease, diabetes mainly – asthma and eczema excluded) living in the Isle of Wight was found to be slightly lower than that of the general population. 17 per cent of these children were reading at a level of at least 28 months below that expected for their age and intelligence, compared with 5.4 per cent in the control group. An important factor in this backwardness appears to be absence from school. Fifteen of the 16 children who were 28 months retarded in reading had been absent from school 70.9 half days in the previous school year, compared with 48.1 for the rest of the children with physical disorders. Absence from school probably also accounts for the slightly lowered intelligence of these children. The loss of confidence which may result from repeated short absences from school was probably as important a factor in the educational retardation of these children as the actual school work missed.

OLCH, D. (1971b) *Journal of Genetic Psychology,* 119, 63–74.

Effects of hemophilia upon intellectual growth and academic achievement

A study of the intellectual and educational functioning of 45 haemophiliac boys and young men, aged 2 to 21 years who were on the files of a major treatment centre in the United States. There was an absence of subjects from the lowest socio-economic level.

Intelligence tended to be in the high average range. Intellectual strengths and weaknesses tended to be related to the children's experiences – they were strong in areas involving manipulation of objects or needing factual knowledge, probably due to time spent making models, reading and watching television when recovering from bleeding episodes, but they were relatively weak in areas needing some understanding of social situations. Academic achievements were generally below the children's level of ability; one-third read below grade level and two-thirds were below grade level in arithmetic.

With increasing age the academic achievements of the haemophiliac child declined in relation to his potential ability. On average the haemophiliac boys missed twice as much schooling as the general school population; often home tutoring was not given as the individual school absences were brief and, on the whole, little special help was provided on the child's return to school. School absences, though, were not clearly related to academic achievements; the main determinants of achievement were intelligence and socio-economic level, certain personality characteristics also playing a part. The author concludes that the haemophiliac child should be given special consideration rather than special schooling. There should be provisions for making up missed school work, even when absences are short.

BAYER, L.M. and HONZIK, M.P. (1976) Springfield, Illinois: Charles C. Thomas.

Children with Congenital Intracardiac Defects

A detailed study of 334 children who underwent surgery for congenital heart defects. The age range was one to 17 years but at the time of surgery most children were between four and eight. 9 per cent of the sample had died. Physical growth, neurological and EEG findings, and psychological and psychiatric records are followed up over several years, and extensive case histories presented for a number of the children. For psychological assessment, a battery of tests was administered to each child before and after surgery, and (for a number of them) at yearly intervals for three years.

Boys' IQs were consistently higher than girls', particularly on the verbal subtest, but the average overall was within the normal range. On the Bender-Gestalt test, a measure of perceptual-motor ability, the children were below average both before and after the operation. Nineteen children were chosen for psychiatric assessment; inquiries were made about family relationships, habits, sleeping and eating, reaction to surgery; projective tests were administered. Before the operation, eight of the 19 were considered to have mild to moderate personality disturbances, but none to be seriously deviant. Six children showed mild reactions to their hospital stay. Of the seven children whose physical status was clearly changed from ill to well by the operation, none showed any inclination to cling to invalidism. It would seem, all in all, that reports of the pathogenic effects of serious physical illness and operations should be reconsidered.

HONZIK, M.P., BUSE, S.T., FITZGERALD, L.H., and COLLART, D.S. (1976) In: BAYER, L.M. and HONZIK, M.P., *Children with Congenital Intracardiac Defects.* Springfield, Illinois: Charles C. Thomas.

Psychologic Development

A battery of tests was administered to children before and after heart surgery. The age range was one to 17 years, with the majority aged four to eight, and socio-economic status was representative of the general population. Tests were given while awaiting surgery in hospital and one month after operation, and a number of the children were followed up for several years. Intelligence scores were within the normal range on both occasions, although girls' verbal scores were lower than boys'. On the Peabody Picture Vocabulary Test girls also scored below average. On the Bender-Gestalt Test scores for all children were rather low both before and after surgery. On the Draw-a-Man Test scores were slightly lowered. Essentially the children's intelligence was shown to be normal, but test results suggested a possible perceptual-motor deficit.

MESSMER, B.J., SCHALLBURGER, U., GATTIKER, R., and SENNING, A. (1976) *Journal of Thoracic and Cardiovascular Surgery,* 72, 4, 495–502.

Psychomotor and intellectual development after deep hypothermia and circulatory arrest in early infancy

A study of the psychomotor and intellectual development of a group of 11 children (five boys, six girls) who had had heart surgery by the method of deep hypothermia and circulatory arrest. Median age at the time of operation was three months, and at the time of the study the children were between 3 and 11 years. They were given a battery of psychological tests, and compared with 11 children who had had major cardiovascular surgery in infancy but without hypothermia and circulatory arrest. The children's height and weight were found to be normal, though they had been seriously underweight before surgery. Average IQ of the whole group fell within the normal range, but three children were retarded, only one of them apparently as a result of the operation. It is concluded that deep hypothermia and circulatory arrest in early infancy are unlikely to have a negative effect of development.

HAEMOPHILIA SOCIETY (1977)

Survey Report

Approximately 1500 questionnaires were distributed to members of the Society and other haemophiliacs; 750 were completed, of which 47 per cent were by respondents under 20. Of the total, 47 per cent considered themselves severely affected, and 80 per cent were receiving treatment – the majority from a haemophilia centre but 13 per cent through home treatment. Over half were being treated at least monthly. 10 per cent were unhappy with the treatment they were getting, 18 per cent with counselling and 32 per cent with advice (or lack of it) on the problem of pain and drug dependence.

Comparing a previous survey and comparing age groups, it was clear that far fewer haemophiliacs are now receiving inadequate education; also, more are now continuing to further education. Respondents were not fully satisfied with their job and education experiences, however; over half would not have chosen their current job if they had not been disabled, and the great majority stated that they felt haemophilia had hindered their prospects.

Respondents were most concerned with pain, crippling, exclusion from heavy work, frequent treatments, and drug dependence, in that order. 22 per cent stated they were reluctant to consider having children, 9 per cent to marry or have sexual relationships, and 20 per cent felt that haemophilia had hindered relationships outside the family.

LUDVIGSSON, J. (1977) *Acta Paediatrica Scandinavica,* 66, 431–7.

Socio-psychological factors and metabolic control in juvenile diabetes

The influence of various factors on metabolic control was studied in 58 diabetic children aged 6 to 17 in Sweden. Social background was average, though parents often found the illness an economic burden. Knowledge about, and attitudes towards, diabetes were estimated among children and parents; 75 per cent of parents but only 38 per cent of older children had adequate knowledge. There was a positive correlation between the knowledge of parents and that of their children and, in the older children, between knowledge and positive attitudes to their illness. Most children had a fairly positive attitude towards it and towards treatment, but this was less marked in children with a late onset.

Intelligence was normal. Out of the 58, seven presented serious psychiatric problems, all but one 'rebellious' teenagers. These had negative attitudes to the illness and poorer control than the rest. 19 per cent had poor diet habits, and this was commoner in the older children. Amount of exercise taken was associated with a positive attitude towards treatment.

MARKOVA, I., LOCKYER, R., and FORBES, C.D. (1977) *Health Bulletin,* 35, 177–82.

Haemophilia: A survey on social issues

A questionnaire survey of 100 patients in Glasgow, of whom nearly half were under 21. About a quarter had been in-patients in hospital within the past two years. At the time of the interview, half the sample had joint symptoms. Although stairs were difficult for many, only one-quarter lived on the ground floor. Much time had been lost from school, especially in severer cases. The more severely affected patients tended to have unskilled jobs, and there was a vicious circle of loss of education, lack of qualifications, unsatisfactory jobs, and dismissals. 46 per cent of patients had had additional financial aid. Better housing is emphasized in the conclusions.

HAKE-IKSE, K., BLACKWOOD, M.J.A., and STEWARD, D.J. (1978) *Developmental Medicine and Child Neurology,* 20, 1, 67–70.

Psychomotor development of infants and children after profound hypothermia during surgery for congenital heart disease

A group of 17 children who had undergone profound hypothermia, and seven siblings as controls, were assessed for neurologic status and cognitive, verbal, social, and motor skills. (The patients had a high incidence of birth problems and other complications which could retard development.) The average Developmental Quotient of the patients was 92.5 and of their siblings 103. A number of children had motor deficit, language delay, or hyperkinesis. Outcome was significantly different in relation to the nature of the cardiac defect. The patients' development was comparable to that reported by other authors for children with cyanotic heart disease who have not undergone surgery.

MYERS-VANDO, R., STEWARD, M.S., FOLKINS, C.H., and HINES, P. (1979) *American Journal of Orthopsychiatry,* 49, 4, 617–25.

The effects of congenital heart disease on cognitive development, illness causality developments, and vulnerability

Twelve Californian children aged 8 to 16, chronically ill with congenital heart disease, were studied; the hypotheses were that they would be at lower levels of cognitive performance on a Piagetian task than well children, that they would be at lower levels of understanding the causes of illness, and that they would demonstrate a greater sense of vulnerability. When their results were compared to those of matched controls, the first and third hypotheses were confirmed.

DICKINSON, D.F. and SAMBROOK, J.E. (1979) *Archives of Disease in Childhood,* 54, 1, 1–6.

Intellectual performance in children after circulatory arrest with profound hypothermia in infancy

Thirty-eight children aged two to eight in Liverpool were assessed for intelligence and social maturity, 22 months to six years after open-heart surgery under profound hypothermia. In all but four cases the operation had been done before two years of age. The mean IQ was 99.2; but there was a wider dispersion of scores about the mean than would be expected, and a significant proportion of survivors showed evidence of intellectual retardation, sometimes dating back to neurological abnormalities noted before the operation.

GATH, A., SMITH, M.A., and BAUM, J.D. (1980) *Archives of Disease in Childhood,* 55, 5, 371–5.

Emotional, behavioural, and educational disorders in diabetic children

The educational and emotional status of 76 children aged 5 to 16 attending a diabetic clinic were assessed, and the relationship with degree of diabetic control and with family circumstances established. The children's schools filled in questionnaires on each child and a matched control; parents were interviewed; diabetic control was assessed by the paediatrician. No significance was found in the duration of illness or family history of diabetes. Psychiatric disorders, overall, were not found significantly more common among the diabetic children than among controls; reading backwardness, however, was significantly more common. Psychiatric disorders and reading backwardness were associated both with poor diabetic control and with adverse family backgrounds.

MARKOVA, I., MACDONALD, K., and FORBES, C. (1980b) *Child: Care, Health and Development,* 6, 2, 101–9.

Integration of haemophilic boys into normal schools

The parents and schools of 36 haemophiliac boys in Scotland were sent questionnaires. Nearly half the parents said that teachers, in spite of their sympathy, did not understand haemophiliacs' problems. There was little communication between the school and the children's hospitals. Absences from school were seen as the main problem by teachers; children away for over six weeks had special tuition, but parents did not find this very helpful. Nevertheless the children did at least averagely well at school. Restrictions on PE varied according to the severity of the illness; a few boys insisted on proving their physical toughness, but no serious accident was reported. 80 per cent of parents would have liked a counselling service, and half of the schools would have liked more information on the illness.

All the teachers supported the integration of the children into normal schools. There remain some problems, however; in particular, lack of communication between school, hospital, and family.

AHNSJÖ, S., HUMBLE, K., LARSSON, Y., SETTERGREN-CARLSON, G., and STERKY, G. (1981) *Acta Paediatrica Scandinavica,* 70, 321–7.

Personality changes and social adjustment during the first three years of diabetes in children

All 64 children over four with newly discovered diabetes at one clinic in Stockholm were studied, together with 30 matched controls. Psychological and social status was assessed, and intelligence tests and Rorschach tests given, soon after discovery of the illness and then three years later. There were no overall significant differences in intellectual or psychological state between the diabetics and controls either on the first or second testing, though diabetics showed an increase in aggressivity, and on the Rorschach they showed an anxiety about health.

O'DOUGHERTY, M., WRIGHT, F.S., GARMEZY, N., LOEWENSON, R.B. and TORRES, F. (1983) *Child Development,* 54, 5, 1129–42.

Later competence and adaptation in infants who survive severe heart defects

Thirty-one school age children who had undergone open-heart surgery for transposition of the great arteries (TGA) were studied, and findings reported in medical detail. Among other results, it was found that (a) although the majority of the children had average intelligence scores, there was a higher than expected proportion of both retarded and gifted children; (b) abnormal neurologic findings were prevalent and a third of the children had abnormal EEG records; (c) children from families experiencing greater life stress had experienced longer duration of hypoxia and more growth failure; (d) socio-economic status and current family stress were both related to intelligence scores and to behavioural ratings; (e) early surgery was associated with better intelligence scores; (f) duration and number of hospitalizations were not related to outcome; (g) a high medical risk score was associated with poorer IQ result; (h) in spite of average to above-average intelligence in 80 per cent of the children, 42 per cent required special tuition for learning or behaviour problems.

SECTION IV

General

Articles summarized in this section are mainly concerned with the treatment and management of children with cardiac conditions, haemophilia, and diabetes. Some give factual information about the conditions. Psychological problems of the child and his or her family, educational and employment problems are discussed by a number of authors.

COOPER, H.
(1959)
South African Medical Journal,
33, 17, 349–52.

Psychological aspects of congenital heart disease

A cardiac clinic should provide psychological assistance for both the child with a congenital heart defect and his or her parents during the pre-operative years. Psychological problems may arise from the child's difficulty in accomplishing physical activities and the consequent inability to keep up with peers or they may stem from faulty parental attitudes produced by feelings of guilt or pathological anxiety. Psychological handling of the child at the actual time of surgery is also discussed.

KATZ, A.H.
(1959)
Social Casework,
40, 321–6.

Some psychosocial problems in hemophilia

The medical problem of haemophilia and the resulting psychological, practical and financial (in the United States) problems for the family are described. Counselling for both the child and the parents is essential – early vocational counselling is particularly important as the haemophiliac adolescent and young adult without a suitable occupation is liable to become dependent and apathetic.

ONGLEY, P.A.
and DUSHANE,
J.W.
(1961)
American Journal of Cardiology, 7,
335–9.

Rehabilitation of the child with congenital heart disease

Treatment and management are discussed for cardiac children: (a) with surgically correctable heart defects; (b) with defects which can be only partially corrected by surgery; (c) who can be helped medically but not surgically; (d) for whom no satisfactory treatment is available at present. General medical management, physical activity and the social and emotional adjustment of the child are considered.

SCHIFF, L.J.
(1964)
Psychosomatics,
5, 6, 362–4.

Emotional problems of diabetic children and their parents

A discussion of parents' problems with guilt, resentment, and over-protection, and children's rebellious attitudes towards the illness when under stress.

INGRAM, G.I.C.
(1965)
British Journal of Clinical Practice,
19, 9, 495–9.

Some problems of social management in haemophilia

Suggestions for meeting problems arising during infancy, school age, and adulthood. At primary school stage teachers should be told in advance about haemophilia, especially about bleeding episodes and unavoidable absences. At secondary level also a preliminary interview with the headmaster or headmistress should be arranged. By this age the boy's response to minor injury will be known and he should take as much part in sport as is compatible with this. Once the boy is old enough to understand his own limitations he should be restricted as little as possible; over-protection may be more harmful than a certain amount of accidental injury.

AGLE, D.P. and MATTSON, A. (1968) *Modern Treatment,* 5, 1, 111–24.

Psychiatric and social care of patients with hereditary hemorrhagic disease

For successful treatment of the haemophiliac patient the physician must both be aware of the emotional stresses that affect the child and his or her family and be able to promote those activities which lead to the most satisfactory adjustment. Aspects discussed by the authors include: the impact of haemophilia on the child and his or her parents; psychiatric syndromes that may occur in haemophiliacs; realistic responses to the illness; parental attitudes; necessity of encouraging judgement and self-reliance in the haemophiliac child; the question of what constitutes a reasonable level of physical activity; psychological management of bleeding episodes; problems of rebellion in adolescence; vocational choice.

WEIL, W.B. Jr. (1968) *New England Journal of Medicine,* 278, 15, 829–31.

Current concepts: juvenile diabetes mellitus

Many problems in diabetes are unresolved and are the subjects of current discussion, including: the relationship between control and late complications in the illness; aetiology; the course of the illness; prescribed or self-selected diet; assessment of control; the age at which a diabetic child should assume responsibility for his or her own management; the purpose and value of summer camps.

KATZ, A.H. (1970c) Springfield, Illinois: Charles C. Thomas.

Hemophilia. A Study in Hope and Reality.

An examination of the social and psychological problems of haemophilia. Based on his own study of 1055 adult haemophiliacs living in the United States and on the research findings of others, the author describes the personal and social characteristics of haemophiliacs and discusses family, educational and employment problems. One chapter is concerned with haemophiliacs' views of themselves and their situation. (See also Katz, 1970a and b (Sections I and III).)

LaHood, B.J. (1970) *Clinical Pediatrics*, 9, 8, 468–71.

Parental attitudes and their influence on the medical management of diabetic adolescents

Juvenile diabetics, previously in good medical control, may experience repeated episodes of acidosis in adolescence. Many factors, including metabolic disturbances, susceptibility to infection and emotional disturbances have been suggested as being responsible. In some cases, though, the diabetic adolescent deliberately sabotages his or her medical regimen, rebelling against over-protection. A social worker or other professional should assess family relationships and management of the condition.

Rizza, C.R. (1970) *Practitioner*, 204, 763–72.

The management of haemophilia

Management and treatment of the haemophiliac patient are discussed. Full use of the specialized haemophilia centres that have been set up throughout the United Kingdom is necessary if the patient is to receive the best treatment. Close collaboration is needed between the general practitioner, hospital, teachers and social workers to ensure that the boy grows up to lead as normal a life as possible with the minimum of crippling. Parents should be given some guidelines by which to judge if bleeds need immediate hospital treatment and they should be encouraged to make plans for the child's education at an early stage.

Younghusband, E., Birchall, D., Davie, R., and Kellmer Pringle, M.L. (Eds) (1970) London: National Bureau for Co-operation in Child Care (now National Children's Bureau).

Living with Handicap

The report of a working party of experts set up under the auspices of the National Children's Bureau to review the needs of handicapped children and the adequacy of the existing services for them. Evidence and information was obtained from professional and voluntary organizations, local authorities and from parents of handicapped children. On the basis of these contributions and their own experiences in various disciplines concerned with handicapped children the working party made detailed recommendations on every aspect of their subject.

HEFFERMAN, A. (1971) In: NOLAND, R.L. (Ed) *Counselling Parents of the Ill and Handicapped.* Springfield, Illinois: Charles C. Thomas, 423–31.

An experiment in group therapy with mothers of diabetic children

Group therapy, over a two-year period, enabled mothers of diabetic children to become more relaxed and confident in their management of the diabetes, gave them increased understanding of their children's reactions to the illness and helped them to handle the children better.

MATTSON, A. (1972) *Pediatrics,* 50, 5, 801–10.

Long-term physical illness in childhood: A challenge to psychosocial adaptation

A detailed examination of the many stresses a chronically ill child and his or her family have to face, and of the ways in which they learn to cope with them. Much depends on the support of the doctor.

LINDE, L.M. and LINDE, S.D. (1973) *American Operating Room Nursing Journal,* 18, 95–99

Emotional factors of pediatric patients in cardiac surgery

Parents' and children's reactions to cardiac surgery are discussed. All parents react with anxiety, part of which is entirely appropriate. Many show grief and anticipatory mourning, making them cling too closely to the child in hospital or else withdraw and fail to visit often enough. Some are hostile to doctors and nurses. For the child, hospitalization is inevitably traumatic, and many regress temporarily. They should be prepared as much as possible for the ordeal of the hospital stay. Nurses' behaviour can make a great difference for both parents and children.

AGLE, D. (1975) *Annals of the New York Academy of Sciences,* 240, 221–5

Psychological factors in hemophilia – the concept of self-care

The specific psychological problems for haemophiliacs regarding activity and aggression are mentioned. Methods, such as home therapy and training in self-hypnosis, which give the haemophiliac a sense of independence, are to be welcomed. One must be aware, however, of some possible drawbacks in home therapy.

AGLE, D.P. and MATTSON, A. (1976) In: HILGARTNER, M. (Ed) *Hemophilia in Childhood,* 137–48.

Psychological complications of hemophilia

Covers the family, stress and the haemophiliac coping behaviour, and management. The future is much brighter for haemophiliacs, due both to improvements in medical technology and to increased understanding of the psychological stresses imposed by the illness.

CRAIG, O. (1977) London: Butterworths. (Especially Chapter 4, 'Behaviour'; Chapter 5, 'Communication and Education', 64–80.)

Childhood Diabetes and its Management

Problems of parent and diabetic child are discussed with humour and insight, as are ways of communicating clearly both at home and at the out-patient clinic. Eleven other chapters cover all aspects of the illness in clear and practical form.

SAUNDERS, A.M. and LAMB, W. (1977) *Journal of Clinical and Child Psychiatry,* 6, 79–82.

A group experience with parents of hemophiliacs: A viable alternative to group therapy

A short-term, directive, problem-solving group for 35 families in Chicago is described. The focus was on information, help with behaviour problems and management, and the parents' own feelings. The main issue became that of setting correct limits to the haemophiliac child's activities.

GREYDANUS, D.E. and HOFMANN, A.D. (1979) *American Journal of Diseases of Childhood,* 33, 10, 1061–6.

Psychological factors in diabetes mellitus

A thorough review of the past 100 years' literature, with special reference to adolescents. The influence of stress and emotion is considered, and its particular relevance to 'brittle diabetes' in adolescence. Research on a specific diabetic personality is summarized and the conclusion drawn that there is no particular 'diabetic personality'. The influence of age of onset is discussed; and the child's understanding of the illness. Recommendations are made for helping adolescents to achieve control and self-care. One hundred references.

HAUSER, S.T. and POLLETS, D. (1979) *Diabetes Care,* 2, 2, 227–32.

Psychological aspects of diabetes mellitus: a critical review

A review article covering four areas: the role of psychological factors in the onset of diabetes; the influence of the environment on it; the psychological adjustment of the diabetic; and the role of the family. Regarding the first question, the authors do not find it proven that diabetes is precipitated by psychological factors. On the second, they do find considerable evidence that emotional factors affect the course of the illness. On the third, they find conflicting findings; a pilot study of their own, however, suggested that diabetic adolescents, particularly boys, had 'lower levels of ego development' than would be expected. On the fourth point studies are few.

LINDE, L.M., KLEIN, N.M., and LEAVITT, P.B. (1979) In: NOSHPITZ, J.D. (Ed) *Basic Handbook of Child Psychiatry.* New York: Basic Books, 447–52.

The child with congenital heart disease

The authors give a background of basic medical knowledge about congenital heart conditions. They review the literature on the psychology of the child with this handicap, and describe ways of supporting child and parents before and during surgery.

ANDERSON, B.J. and AUSLANDER, W.F. (1980) *Diabetes Care,* 3, 6, 696–702.

Research on diabetes management and the family: a critique

A review article focusing on discussions of the relation of the whole family to a member with juvenile diabetes. Two consistent findings emerge: parental attitudes towards the treatment regime are inextricable from their general child-rearing attitudes; and low stress is associated with good control. Methodological faults are pointed out, and directions for future research suggested.

DUNN, S.M. and TURTLE, J.R. (1981) *Diabetes Care,* 4, 6, 640–6.

The myth of the diabetic personality

Forty years of studies on the 'diabetic personality' are reviewed, and the conclusion reached that there is no serious evidence for its existence. Samples of diabetic adolescents in particular have been biased, and control groups inadequate. Diabetics respond to their illness in a multitude of different ways.

EGLI, H. and INWOOD, M.J. (Eds) (1981) Munich: Karger.

The Haemophiliac in the Eighties

Proceedings of the First International Haemophilia Conference at Bonn. Includes care and management, haemophiliacs' organizations, reports from 35 countries, the haemophiliac yesterday and today, a review of psychosocial adjustment, and a number of medical papers.

KOSUB, S.M. and CERRETO, M.C. (1981) *Social Work in Health Care,* 6, 4, 91–101.

Juvenile diabetes: current trends in psychosocial research

A review article assessing the literature on juvenile diabetes and psychological stress. Research has so far tended to focus either on the 'diabetic personality', on family interactions, or on environmental stress such as bereavement. The limitations of each approach are discussed. It is suggested that multiple interacting causes are involved and that predisposition, stress, and environment should be seen as all influencing one another.

TATTERSALL, R.B. and LOWE, J. (1981) *Diabetologia,* 20, 517–23.

Diabetes in adolescence

A consideration of the extra problems of independence and self-esteem imposed by adolescence on the diabetic youngster. Recommendations for management are made: transfer to the adults' clinic, change of doctor and possibly regime, coping with teenage diet conventions, caring for the 'brittle' diabetic, the questions of alcohol and sex. Teenagers should be treated with consideration, and helped to talk out any family problems.

FISHER, E.B., DELAMATER, A.M., BERTELSON, A.D., and KIRKLEY, B.G. (1982) *Journal of Consulting and Clinical Psychology,* 50, 6, 993–1003.

Psychological factors in diabetes and its treatment

An extensive review of recent findings on aetiology, psychological adjustment, family dynamics, and counselling. Research should clarify the role of stress and focus on psychological factors related to metabolic control, and also assess the value of help offered. Ninety-seven references.

JOHNSON, S.B. and ROSENBLOOM, A.L. (1982) *Psychiatric Clinics of North America,* 5, 2, 357–69.

Behavioral aspects of diabetes mellitus in childhood and adolescence

The specific problems of juvenile diabetes are discussed; the factors, such as age, stress, family patterns, and doctor–patient relationship, that affect its management; and the role of the psychiatrist or psychologist.

LINDE, L.M. (1982) *Psychiatric Clinics of North America,* 5, 2, 399–406.

Psychiatric aspects of congenital heart disease

A discussion of the psychological factors involved – breathing and feeding difficulties, restrictions – for the child with a cardiac handicap, the experience of hospital and operation, and the anxieties and problems of the parents.

BLOOM, A. (1983) British Diabetic Association.

Life with Diabetes

An illustrated booklet covering practical points in an easy-to-read format.

BRADBURY, A.J. and SMITH, C.S. (1983) *Archives of Disease in Childhood,* 58, 9, 692–6.

An assessment of the diabetic knowledge of school teachers

Ninety-seven primary and secondary school teachers of diabetic pupils completed questionnaires to assess their knowledge of the illness. Only a quarter showed a reasonably adequate knowledge (14 out of 18 questions correct), and the average score was 10.4. Thirty-five teachers failed to complete the questionnaire, and these may have had an even more inadequate knowledge. Teachers' information had come chiefly from the children and their parents rather than from medical or nursing personnel. Nearly all expressed a wish for more information.

BRITISH DIABETIC ASSOCIATION (1983)

The Diabetic Handbook

The Association's 27 brief leaflets bound together in one book. Subjects covered include treatment, diet, childhood and adolescence, school, social services, employment, exercise and sport.

KRAUSER, K.L. and MADDEN, P.B. (1983) *Nursing Clinics of North America,* 18, 4, 749–62.

The child with diabetes mellitus

An examination of the needs of the diabetic child at each age level; how to provide some autonomy and understanding of the illness, and avoid unnecessary conflict. Diet, exercise, testing and injections, both at school and at home, are discussed in relation to the child's emotional needs.

CHEST, HEART AND STROKE ASSOCIATION (1984) Leaflet H.155.

Congenital Heart Disease

Basic information for parents about congenital heart defects. Advice on how to prepare the child for diagnostic tests or surgery is also given.

Author Index

Ack, M., Miller, I. and Weil, W.B. Jr. (1961) 47
Agle, D.P. (1964) 11, (1975) 63
Agle, D.P. and Mattson, A. (1968) 61, (1976) 64
Ahnsjö, S., Humble, K., Larsson, Y., Settergren-Carlson, G. and Sterky, G. (1981) 58
Aisenberg, R.B., Wolff, P.H., Rosenthal, A. and Nadas, A.S. (1973) 19
Allen, A.A., Tennen, H., McGrade, B.J., Affleck, G. and Ratzan, S. (1984) 41
Anderson, B.J. and Auslander, W.F. (1980) 65
Anderson, B.J., Miller, J.P., Auslander, W.F. and Santiago, J.V. (1981) 39
Apley, J., Barbour, R.F. and Westmacott, I. (1967) 32

Baker, L., Minuchin, S., Milman, S., Liebman, R. and Todd, T. (1975) 36
Bayer, L.M. and Honzik, M.P. (1976) 53
Birkbeck, J.A., Klonoff, H. and McTaggart, A.H. (1968) 14
Bloom, A. (1983) 67
Boon, A.R. (1972) 34
Börner, S. and Steinhausen, H.C. (1977) 37
Bradbury, A.J. and Smith, C.S. (1983) 67
British Diabetic Association (1983) 67
Bronks, I.G. and Blackburn, E.K. (1968) 48
Browne, W.J., Mally, M.A. and Kane, R.P. (1960) 7

Chest, Heart and Stroke Association (1984) 68
Cooper, H. (1959) 60
Craig, O. (1977) 64
Crain, A.J., Sussman, M.B. and Weil, W.B. Jr. (1966a and b) 32

Danowski, T.S. (1963) 9
Delbridge, L. (1975) 37
Del Vecchio, F.A. (1971) 17
Dickinson, D.F. and Sambrook, J.E. (1979) 57
Drash, P.W. and Money, J. (1968) 49
Dunn, S.M. and Turtle, J.R. (1981) 65

Egli, H. and Inwood, M.J. (Eds.) (1981) 66
Etzwiler, D.D. and Sines, L.K. (1962) 8

Fällström, K. (1974) 19

Feldt, R.H., Ewart, J.C., Stickler, G.B. and Weidman, W.H. (1969) 49
Fisher, E.B., Delamater, A.M., Bertelson, A.D. and Kirkley, B.G. (1982) 66

Gabriel, H.P. and Danilowicz, D. (1978) 22
Garlinghouse, J. and Sharp, L.J. (1968) 14
Garson, A., Scott Benson, R., Ivler, L. and Patton, C. (1978) 38
Garson, M.D., Williams, R.B. and Reckless, J. (1974) 20
Gath, A., Smith, M.A. and Baum, J.D. (1980) 57
Glaser, H.H., Harrison, G.S., and Lynn, D.B. (1964) 31
Goldy, F.B. and Katz, A.H. (1963) 9
Graham, P. and Rutter, M. (1970) 16
Greydanus, D.E. and Hofmann, A.D. (1979) 64
Grobler, T. (1981) 24

Haemophilia Society (1977) 54
Hake-Ikse, K., Blackwood, M.J.A. and Steward, D.J. (1978) 56
Hauser, S.T. and Pollets, D. (1979) 65
Hefferman, A. (1971) 63
Honzik, M.P., Buse, S.T., Fitzgerald, L.H. and Collart, D.S. (1976) 54
Honzik, M.P., Collart, D.S., Robinson, S.J. and Finley, K.H. (1969) 50

Ingram, G.I.C. (1965) 60

Johnson, S.B. and Rosenbloom, A.L. (1982) 67

Katz, A.H. (1959) 60, (1963) 9, (1970a) 16, (1970b) 51, (1970c) 61
Kinmonth, A., Lindsay, M.K.M. and Baum, J.D. (1983) 25
Kitchen, L.W. (1978) 22
Klein, R.H. and Nimorwicz, P. (1982) 40
Koski, M-L., Ahlas, A. and Kumento, A. (1976) 37
Kosub, S.M. and Cerreto, M.C. (1981) 66
Krauser, K.L. and Madden, P.B. (1983) 68
Kronenfeld, J.K. and Ory, M.G. (1981) 40
Krones, P.D. (1970) 16
Kupst, M.J., Blatterbauer, S., Westman, J., Schulman, J.L. and Paul, M.H. (1977) 38

LaHood, B.J. (1970) 62
Landtman, B., Valanne, E.H. and Aukee, M. (1968) 15
Landtman, B., Valanne, E.H., Pentti, R. and Aukee, M. (1960) 7
Lavigne, J.V., Traisman, H.S., Marr, T.J. and Chasnoff, I.J. (1982) 25
Leaverton, D.R., White, C.A., McCormick, C.R., Perrin Smith, M.S. and Sheikholislam, B. (1980) 24
Linde, L.M. (1982) 67
Linde, L.M. and Linde, S.D. (1973) 63
Linde, L.M., Klein, N.M. and Leavitt, P.B. (1979) 65
Linde, L.M., Rasof, B. and Dunn, O.J. (1970) 16
Linde, L.M., Rasof, B., Dunn, O.J. and Rabb, E. (1966) 12
Ludvigsson, J. (1977) 55

Madden, N.A., Terrizzi, J. and Friedman, S.B. (1982) 41
Markova, I., and Forbes, C. (1979) 38
Markova, I., Lockyer, R. and Forbes, C.D. (1977) 56
Markova, I., Macdonald, K. and Forbes, C. (1980a) 39, (1980b) 57
Mattson, A. (1972) 63
Mattson, A. and Gross, S. (1966) 12
Maxwell, G.M. and Gane, S. (1962) 31
Meijer, A. (1980) 39

Messmer, B.J., Schallburger, U., Gattiker, R. and Senning, A. (1976) 54
Meyers, R.D. *et al.* (1972) 34
Myers-Vando, R., Steward, M.S., Folkins, C.H. and Hines, P. (1979) 56

Neuhaus, E.C. (1958) 6

O'Dougherty, M., Wright, F.S., Garmezy, N., Loewenson, R.B. and Torres, F. (1983) 58
Offord, D.R. and Aponte, J.F. (1967) 33
Offord, D.R., Cross, L.A., Andrews, E.J. and Aponte, J.F. (1972) 35
Olatawura, M.O. (1972) 18
Olch, D. (1971a) 17, (1971b) 52
Ongley, P.A. and Dushane, J.W. (1961) 60

Rasof, B., Linde, L.M. and Dunn, O.J. (1967) 47
Reed, M.K. (1959) 6
Rizza, C.R. (1970) 62

Salk, L., Hilgartner, M. and Granich, B. (1972) 35
Saunders, A.M. and Lamb, W. (1977) 64
Schiff, L.J. (1964) 60
Silbert, A., Wolff, P.H., Mayer, B., Rosenthal, A. and Nadas, A.S. (1969) 50
Simonds, J.F. (1976/7) 21, (1977) 22
Simonds, J., Goldstein, D., Walker, B. and Rawlings, S. (1981) 24
Soulier, J.P. and Josso, F. (Eds) (1966) 47
Stein, S.P. and Charles, E.S. (1971) 18, (1975) 21
Steinhausen, H.C. (1976) 21
Sterky, G. (1963) 10
Sullivan, B.-J. (1978) 23, (1979) 23
Swift, C.R. and Seidman, F.L. (1964) 11
Swift, C.R., Seidman, F.L., and Stein, H. (1967) 13

Tattersall, R.B. and Lowe, J. (1981) 66
Teitz, W. and Vidmar, J.T. (1972) 18
Treuting, T.F. (1962) 8

Watson, A. (1972) 36
Weil, W.B. Jr. (1968) 61
Weil, W.B. Jr. and Ack, M. (1964) 47
Weil, W.B. Jr and Sussman, M.B. (1967) 14

Younghusband, E., Birchall, D., Davie, R. and Kellmer Pringle, M.L. (Eds) (1970) 62
Yule, W. and Rutter, M. (1970) 52